Management of An Unconscious Pediatric Patient

Dr. Benjamin Alli is a Sakellarides Professor of Medicine & Surgery and the Chancellor of
The Royal College of Physicians and Surgeons of the United States of America.

Published By: **Elite Exclusivity**
Edited By: **Mugheer Ahmad**

Introduction By: Dr. Christopher W. Smithmyer

Elite exclusivity

Dysart Detroit Dallas

Send all Inquiries to: Info@EliteExclusivity.com and
EliteExclusivityPR@gmail.com

First Edition 2023

ISBN Paperback 978-1-952651-04-5
ISBN Hardback: 978-1-952651-11-3
ISBN Digital: 978-1-952651-05-2

Printed in the United States of America

Table of Contents

Introduction

The question is one of the simplest forms of human learning. As a child, we begin with asking "why?" about the world around us. As we age, the questions become more complex and the answers, likewise, lead us to many more questions. In the Post-Covid era, talking heads and political pundits oft repeat the mantra, "Trust the Science;" however, this shows the ignorance of the "Press Class" within our society. Part of science is always questioning. Question the methods. Question the results. Question the data. Question every aspect of the field until a light has been shined on every nook, every cranny. Only then will we have the wisdom to understand the knowledge which we have arrived at.

Dr. Benjamin Alli is one of the most lettered men in the world. He has dedicated his life to the pursuit of a greater knowledge of the medical field. Now in his dotage, Dr. Alli is giving back to the world more than he has taken from it by presenting this text in its present form. Rather than adapt the text to wrought prose as is common in "pulp" books, Dr. Alli has chosen to follow a question/answer format for this book. The data presented is quite detailed, running the spectrum of pediatric issues that may be faced. Dr. Alli addresses how things were done, how they are done, and how they will be done in the magnum examination of the field.

Though ten questions only scratch the surface of the knowledge that can be gained through a study of pediatric medicine, they are supremely focused to bring the field into a better light. Each answer pointed to its necessary end, making this a quick read for those who are on the go. While relatively short by most standards, this pocketbook is an excellent addition to any library, especially in this First edition, not corrupted by editorial changes, looking at the raw knowledge of one of the greatest minds in the field. Enjoy and recognize that the field is always expanding- and every one of us lives or has lived in this field.

EMERGENCY TREATMENT AND APPROACH TO THE MANAGEMENT OF AN UNCONSCIOUS PEDIATRIC PATIENT

Unconscious pediatric patients are different from unconscious adult patients in several ways. There are many differences between the causes, communication, and caregivers.

The causes of unconsciousness in pediatric patients are often different from those in adults. In children, common causes of unconsciousness include head injuries, seizures, choking, infections, and poisoning. In contrast, adults are more likely to experience unconsciousness due to heart attacks, strokes, and drug overdoses.

Children's bodies and organs are still developing, so their anatomy and physiology differ from those of adults. As a result, they may require different doses of medication, different medical equipment, and different approaches to resuscitation.

Unconscious pediatric patients cannot communicate their symptoms and medical history, so healthcare providers must rely on other sources of information, such as family members or medical records. Also, they often require emotional support from their families and caregivers. Healthcare providers must consider the child's developmental stage and provide age-appropriate emotional support.

Caregivers play a critical role in the care of unconscious pediatric patients. Healthcare providers must communicate effectively with caregivers and involve them in the decision-making process.

Healthcare providers should have specialized training and experience in the care of unconscious pediatric patients to provide the best possible care and outcomes.

What is generally thought of as the guidelines in an unfortunate scenario as in the title?

In the event of an unconscious pediatric patient, immediately call for emergency medical services. Time is crucial in such situations, and the patient's life may depend on how quickly they receive medical attention.

Try to arouse the child by tapping on their shoulders or calling out their name. If the child does not respond, the airway should be checked for any obstructions.

If the child is not breathing, begin cardiopulmonary resuscitation (CPR). If the child has a pulse but is not breathing, perform rescue breathing. If the child does not have a pulse, perform CPR with chest compressions and rescue breathing.

Determine if there are any obvious signs of trauma or injury, such as bleeding or fractures. If there are, address them appropriately while continuing to provide medical attention.

Monitor the child's vital signs, including their blood pressure, heart rate, and oxygen saturation levels, if possible.

If the child has a history of seizures, administer any prescribed medication to control seizures.

Transport to the hospital: Once the child's condition is stabilized, they should be transported to the nearest hospital for further evaluation and treatment.

These steps are considered a general guideline, but the approach varies depending on the specific situation. Proper training and certification in pediatric emergency care to provide effective treatment in these situations is especially important.

Consider aspects of the title not always considered.

Unconsciousness or coma may be caused broadly by two types of lesions or processes:

1. Those that affect the reticular formation of the brain stem, which may also involve the centersof respiration and circulation control, and
2. Those that affect the brain diffusely, including Central nervous system lesions, systemic infections, and toxic or metabolic disturbances.

For practical purposes, in emergencies, comatose patients may be classified into three pathophysiologic categories.

1. Metabolic coma that is immediately treatable.
2. Rapidly progressive supratentorial or sub-tectorial masses or destructive lesions, and
3. Non-progressive coma, including psychogenic coma.

As a rule, metabolic causes of coma lead to a symmetrical involvement, while focalabnormalities suggest intracranial mass lesions, particularly when brainstem abnormalities are present.

The management of an unconscious patient falls arbitrarily into two phases in the acute phase. The emergency treatment is mainly to promptly stabilize the patient through supportivetherapy and protect him from further damage. In this phase, treatment precedes diagnosis. In the second phase, which may overlap the first, detailed history-taking, and evaluation is doneto establish the cause of the problem and take measures to deal with potential complications of prolonged unconsciousness.

The Glasgow Coma Scale is important for emergent neurologic assessment of the unconscious patient and for planning management. It is based on bed side examination directed at measuring the arousal and responsiveness of the patient. It allows staging by serial examination of eye-opening, verbal, and best motor responses. A score of <9 suggeststhat the patient has severe brain dysfunction and airway support is a priority. Intracranial pressure and invasive hemodynamic monitoring are required.

Emergency treatment of an unconscious child involves the followingsteps and procedures:

1) Intermediate resuscitation and stabilization of the patient, including positioning,maintaining the airway, and ensuring breathing and adequate circulation.

2) Administration of glucose, 2ml of 25% dextrose/ Kg to correct possible hypoglycemia.

3) Treatment of seizures, if any, by phenobarbitone or phenytoin.

4) Quick gathering of information initially about the symptoms and circumstances leading to and since unconsciousness relevant to the patient's age. This is followed later, as time allows, by detailed history-taking, including drugs, travel, past, ard family history.

5) Rapid physical examination and neurological assessment noting vital signs, BP, andinjury, Glasgow Coma Scale, pallor, cyanosis, jaundice, hydration status, odor, any rashes or petechiae, pupil size and reactions, eye movements, reflexes, fundus examination, head circumference. ECG is taken, and pulse oximetry is done.
6) Initial investigations included full blood count,

plasma glucose, serum electrolytes, urea, calcium, phosphate, magnesium, ammonia, blood gases, and coagulation screen. Urine testing, including destrostix (a rapid test for the determination of blood sugar) and microscopy, is carried out. CT Head and US Head may be urgently needed. X-ray chest (portable) is done.

Cases of Traumatic injuries involving the head and other systems shouldbe evaluated by a team, including a pediatric surgeon. Hypotension in such patients suggestssystemic trauma and control of shock is urgently required.

If the child has a major abdominal or thoracic injury requiring operative intervention, this gets priority over most head injuries.

- In a child with isolated head trauma, if the x-ray rules out acutely life-threateningchest injuries, neurosurgical intervention after a CT scan of the head takes priority.

- In a comatose child with no history of trauma, neurosurgical evaluation and intervention may still be required to rule out spontaneous intracerebral hemorrhage or brain tumors. The pupils are acutely unequal or unreactive. This is highly suggestive of a progressivemass lesion and requires emergency treatment of an impending herniation.

- In a child with fever or meningism, when meningitis is considered a possibility, LP should be performed (after CT head). Antibiotics are started promptly, sometimes even prior to LP.

- In case of poisoning, measures are taken to hasten the removal of poison from the blood andtissues. The techniques used include emesis and gastric suctioning using activated charcoal, forced diuresis with urinary pH control (ion trapping), peritoneal or hemodialysis, hemoperfusion, and exchange transfusion. Specific drug antibodies/antidotes are available for certain poisons and are given accordingly.

DIAGNOSTIC WORK UP AND FURTHER MANAGEMENT

The following causes have been usually excluded by initial history and investigations. A detailed history-taking and investigation plan are executed to establish the diagnosis.

- Trauma to the head and other systems.
- Drowning
- Burn
- Diabetic ketoacidosis
- Other metabolic causes of coma include hypoxia, hypoglycemia, abnormalities ofelectrolytes, acidosis, alkalosis, uremia, hepatic failure, hyperammonemia, and hyperosmolar states.
- Cardiovascular accident
- Infections

Other investigations to be Carried Out Were Indicated:

- Septic screen to exclude infections (bacterial, fungal, and protozoal)
- Lumbar puncture, if not already done a CSF studies
- Virologic studies on blood and CSF
- Toxicological screen for excluding poisoning with Alcohol, Barbiturates, Benzodiazepines, Salicylates opiates, Carbon monoxide, Paracetamol, Lead Iron, Anticonvulsants, Anticholinergics, Antidepressants, and Organophosphates.
- X-ray of chest, skull, skeletal
- Tests for other metabolic causes:
- Liver function tests and coagulation profile
  - ❖ Lactate, Pyruvate, T4, TSH

    - Tuberculin test
- Liver-spleen radionuclide scan
- MRI, if indicated

Supportive Investigations and Monitoring

- ECG and BP monitoring
- Blood osmolality
- EEG – Continuous
- ICP/CCP- mean pressure, pulse pressure
- Visual evoked potentials
- Brain stem evoked potential

ANSWERS TO QUESTION-2

MATERNAL DEATH- CAUSES AND PREVENTION

Maternal death and its causes vary from one country to another in incidence. Though many reductions have been achieved in maternal mortality (for example, from 83/100,000 livebirths to 7.4 in the USA), problems remain worldwide.

Five important problems associated with maternal morbidity and mortality are:

1. Malnutrition
2. Hypertension
3. Antepartum Hemorrhage
4. Diabetes mellitus
5. Abortion

Malnutrition

Malnutrition that occurs due to poverty or inadequate intake is an important direct and indirect cause of maternal and infant morbidity and mortality. Chronic malnutrition prior to pregnancy, particularly if starting early during childhood, may result in low body weight and decreased body stores for the fetus, as well as reduced immunity. It also may cause a contracted pelvis leading to cephalopelvic disproportion problems during delivery.

Various nutritional deficiencies are observed more often during pregnancy. Anemia is a common disease fining in women of lower socio-economic class, particularly in those areaswhere other associated factors like malaria, hookworm infestation, tuberculosis, and gastrointestinal diseases co-exist. Deficiency of iron with or without folic acid deficiency iscommon. Insufficient weight gain during pregnancy due to inadequate nutrition or illnessesleads to compromised fetal and maternal health and, consequently, increased morbidity and mortality.

Preeclampsia and Eclampsia:

It is necessary to provide explicit health and nutrition advice to girls in schools and in thepopulation, and in the antenatal clinics in hospitals.

Provide a diet sufficient in calories and all the nutrients supplemented with iron in the formof 30mg of ferrous gluconate on sulfate plus 1mg of folic acid daily. A weight gain of 1 to 2kg during the first trimester and then almost 0.5kg each week thereafter should be optimal.

Early detection of diseases and effective treatment is a must.

HYPERTENSION

Although the incidence of serious complications associated with hypertension has greatly reduced because of advancements in perinatal care, they remain a significant cause of maternaland fetal morbidity and mortality.

From five to ten percent of pregnancies are complicated by hypertensive disease. American College of Obstetricians and Gynecologists classify hypertensive disorder or pregnancy intoPreeclampsia and eclampsia chronic hypertension, chronic hypertension with superimposed preeclampsia and eclampsia, and late transient hypertension.

Hypertension during pregnancy is a rise of 30mm Hg in systolic or 15mm Hg in morediastolic pressure or a Bp> 140/90.

Preeclampsia and Eclampsia:

Most commonly, preeclampsia affects women at both extremes of reproductive age but occurspredominantly in primigravida during the second half of pregnancy. In multigravidas, it is more commonly associated with plural gestation, fetal hydrops, hydatidiform mole, and diabetes mellitus with chronic hypertension.

Preeclampsia is characterized by the development of hypertension, proteinuria, extracellular fluid retention, and facial or hand edema. Rapid weight gain occurs (1.36kg per week). Proteinuria is >300mg of protein in 24 hours or a protein concentration of 1 g/l in twoor more random samples collected at least 6 hours apart. At levels of 5gm or more / within 24 hours, ŧis severe.

Two fundamental pathologic processes are preeclampsia are generalized small artery spasmsand increased capillary permeability.

The –roll over‖ test measuring BP may identify the potential development of preeclampsia. Symptoms such as headache, severe epigastric pain, hyperreflexia, and hemoconcentrationusually signal the development of eclampsia when seizures occur.

Completions of preeclampsia and eclampsia include intrauterine growth retardation, abruptioplacentae, cerebrovascular accidents, acute renal failure, cardiac failure, hemolysis, DIC, andhepatic failure. HELLP syndrome occurs with abnormal liver enzymes and low platelet count.

If management at the home of incipient pre-eclampsia or with bed rest in the left lateral recumbentposition does not suffice, hospitalization is indicated for close monitoring and necessary treatment and delivery or Caesarian section when indicated.

Magnesium sulfate is the drug of choice for preventing and treating convulsions (4gm IV slowly followed by 1g/hr.). Hydralazine is the antihypertensive of choice given in 019mg IVdoses at 15-20 minutes intervals until diastolic pressure approaches 90mmHG.

Chronic Hypertensive Disease

It is usually seen in multigravidas and is present before pregnancy (as essential hypertension)or before the 2nd half of gestation. Superimposed preeclampsia or eclampsia is a serious complication and leads to significant fetal and maternal morbidity and mortality. Early delivery may be the best management.

If hypertension doesn't 't responds to the conservative measure of antihypertensives such as methyldopa may be tried IV hydralazine, and intensive care management will be requiredto save the mother and the child from complications.

ANTEPARTUM HAEMORRHAGE

Significant vaginal bleeding during the third trimester of pregnancy can be a life-threateningproblem. It may be caused by placenta previa and abruptio placentae.

Placenta previa is characterized by painless vaginal bleeding when the bleeding is brightenedred, in which case it is rare to find uterine contractions, fetal distress, or hypertension. In the case of abruptio placentae, there is pain and uterine hyperreactivity, and tenderness with fetal distress. Hypertension and acute renal failure may be present.

Following hospitalization, therapy with IV fluids started, and a US examination was done to localize the placenta.

Both placenta previa and abruptio placentae are associated with multiparity and advancingmaternal age. In the case of abruptio placentae, another associated condition may be abdominal trauma. The short umbilical cord, vena cava compression, uterine anomaly or tumor, and malnutrition

Prevention of mortality due to antepartum hemorrhage involves family planning advice, ensuring optimal health and nutrition before conception and during pregnancy, and regularantenatal checkups.

DIABETES MELLITUS DURING PREGNANCY

The occurrence of diabetes-associated fetal and maternal mortality is greatly decreased sinceinsulin use though the incidence of diabetes associated with pregnancy has increased. Diabetes, whether preexisting or gestational, contributes to morbidity. Diabetic pregnancy isassociated with an increased incidence of preeclampsia (about 4 times higher), infection, large-sized babies, hydramnios, and postpartum hemorrhage.

Risk factors for gestational diabetes include maternal age of 25 years or older, obesity, familyhistory of diabetes in a first-degree relative, history of pregnancy with stillbirth or infant weighing> 4000 g, and previous infant with congenital anomalies.

Indications for screening for diabetes prior to 24 weeks of gestation include previous gestational diabetes, previous large for gestational age baby, hydramnios, and glycosuria.Polyuria or polydipsia and recurrent urinary or vaginal infections.

A diabetes test is considered abnormal if a screening test with 50gm glucose PO gives a venous plasma glucose level of 140 mg/dl after 1hr or if 3hrs glucose tolerance test (GTT) after 100gm glucose PO gives any two elevated levels.

Cases of gestational diabetes, who have a normal fasting blood glucose level but abnormal GTT, are generally treated by diet alone. This consists of 30-35kcal/ kg/day of actual body weight consisting of 35 to 40 percent of the calories as carbohydrates. 30-35% as proteins and the reaming calories as fat. Regular monitoring and antenatal visit are arranged. Insulin therapy is initiated if the fasting level exceeds 105 mg/dl or the 2hour postprandial value is above120mg/dl on two or more occasions with a 2-week interval. If fetal macrosomia is found at term Caesarian is done.

ABORTION

Abortion is the delivery or loss of the product of conception before the 20th week of pregnancy. Itmay be spontaneous or induced. The incidence of spontaneous abortion is about 20%.

Since in 90% of spontaneous abortions, the fetus is either absent (blighted ova) or is grosslymalformed, and in another 5%, chromosomal abnormalities are found, spontaneous abortion may be regarded as a natural purposeful rejection.

Maternal disease responsible includes acute and chronic infections, chronic diseases, severegeneral malnutrition, endocrine diseases, and antigenic incompatibilities between sexual partners. Other maternal factors may be anomalies of the reproductive tract and tumors. Incompetent cervix, or laparotomy during pregnancy.

Environmental causes leading to abortion include radiation, cytotoxic and other drugs and chemicals affecting the mother or the fetus resulting in congenital malformation and abortion. A woman who had three or more spontaneous abortions is said to have a behavioral abortion.

Threatened Abortion.

Only one-half of all cases go on to abort regardless of treatment. Bed rest and mild sedationmay be successful. Persistent, significant bleeding and pain are treated by hospitalization andpossible termination of pregnancy.

Missed Abortion.

This could cause maternal blood coagulopathy and massive bleeding, particularly if the fetus dies during the second trimester of pregnancy. Evacuation of the uterus therapeutically is doneby IV oxytocin or prostaglandin E2 vaginal suppositories.

Septic Abortion.

It usually occurs after an induced abortion by an untrained person. Septicemia and shockmay occur with grave consequences. Genital infections in the mother with several microorganisms are predisposing factors. Appropriate antibiotic treatment is to be carriedout on an emergency basis after the necessary septic workup.

Prevention.

Prevention of Abortion-related death involves the planning of pregnancy, regular antenatalvisits, avoiding environmental causes, diagnosing, and treating any illness prior to conception or early in pregnancy, and use of legal abortion facilities.

ANSWER TO QUESTION-3

DEVELOPMENT OF MATERNAL HEALTH SERVICES

The goals for maternal health services are the birth of a healthy baby without complications in the mother, the development of the basis for strong bonding between mother and infant, and healthy life for her family as well as for herself after the childbearing year's end. The goals may, however, differ in different societies, both in quantitative and qualitative terms.

In a rational world, health services would be based on the need, prevalence, and impact of health problems of the population and the knowledge base and resources available for successful intervention. The present health status in terms of demographic and morbidity data, the structure of the existing healthcare systems as well as the experience of the past decades in the implementation of the services are influential determinants in future planning. This, coupled with the expectations of society in the context of total socio-economic development, should help shape the future frames of the programmers. In Kuwait, as basic health services are provided almost free, the implementation requires only education and motivation.

MATERNAL HEALTH SERVICES FOR THE PRECONCEPTION STAGE

This should address the following issues:

1. The general health status of the would-be mothers is to be improved. Growth and development during childhood should be the starting point to prepare for a healthyyoung adult. An integrated optimal child health service is a

prerequisite.

2. Education of the girls in schools and later in community groups about reproductivephysiology and anatomy. Sex education and basic knowledge about sexually transmitted diseases (STDs), including HIV, should be imparted through formal as well as informal teaching.
3. Adolescent Health Clinics to manage such problems related to menstruation,social interaction, and prevention of STDs.
4. Knowledge of family planning, safe motherhood, and baby care should be provided through clinics, lectures, leaflets, and mass media. Consanguinity and heredity factors need to be explained.
5. The preconception of health checkups in specialized clinics focuses on the following:
   - Physical examination to rule out or detect any abnormalities, weight, height, BP,and general nutritional status to be evaluated.
   - Any family history of hereditary diseases and Genetic death counseling shouldbe offered if any risk is suspected.
   - Any past illness which may reduce the potential of safe motherhood.
   - Adequate treatment is needed.
   - Psychosocial family atmosphere, the support provided.
   - A schedule of screening is to be followed for detecting any local or systemic disease like diabetes, hypertension, sexually transmitted diseases, and anemia ornutritional deficiencies.
   - Pap smear
   - Rubella immunization (If not already given) at least 3 months prior to conception.

6. High-risk groups are to be detected and provided specialized care, including social support. These individuals are characterized by the inability to plan, to consider the needs of others (family and friends) and have low self-esteem and defeatist attitudes. They may have a family history of hereditary or congenital diseases, still births, or abortions. Those with chronic systemic disease need regular management.
   A social or legal system can be developed to encourage all would-be mothers to go at least once for preconception checkups and necessary follow-ups, with feedback from the regional or local maternity clinics, and when they conceive, this information is referred to. Alternatively, pre-conception health care should be available to all would-be mothers, keeping confidentiality in mind.

ANTENANTAL HEALTH SERVICES

Planned development in the whole state of operation is to be considered in relation to thepopulation density, fertility rate, and socio-economic factors. This should preferably be integrated with Family Medicine and structured in a three-tier system – Primary Clinics,Specialized Clinics, and Tertiary Referral Hospitals.

Primary Clinics should be responsible under the care of trained family physicians to evaluatethe health status of the pregnant lady from physical and psychosocial aspects. The preconception check-up records should be referred to. A thorough medical and obstetric examination followed by initial laboratory tests and pulse-echo sonography is performed.

The objectives are:

1. Ascertain the health status of the mother.

2. Confirm a pregnancy and establish gestational age. A review at each subsequent visitis desired so that untoward events such as premature labor-the principal cause of perinatal death, premature rupture of fetal membrane, IU growth retardation, and post-maturity may be avoided or appropriately treated. Fetal development is regularly monitored at each visit, and the expected date of confinement is established.

3. A Scoring system can be devised and used to know high-risk pregnant groups needing specialized care, including detailed investigations and close monitoring

4. Initial ante mental laboratory tests should include the following:
    - Blood type and Rh factor
    - Antibody screen for sensitization
    - Hemoglobin and hematocrit (repeated at 24 weeks and term)
    - Sickle cell screen, when indicated
    - Rubella tire
    - Hepatitis B screening (HBs Ag)
    - Serology testing with VDRL OR RPR
    - If positive, FTA-ABS is performed
    - Urinalysis and culture (Urinalysis for protein and glucose repeated at eachvisit)
    - Pap smear
    - Cervical culture for gonorrhea (repeat near term)
    - Plasma glucose
    - Screening for gestational diabetes with

plasma glucose 1hr after 50g oral glucose load was performed at the initial visit and again at 24-28 weeks in at-risk women. If the venous plasma glucose level is 140/mg dl or above, a 100g 3-hour glucose tolerance test is performed.

5. Prenatal detection of genetic abnormalities is required for Neutral tube defects, Down syndrome, Hemophilia, Tay Sech 's Disease, and Other chromosomal and biochemical abnormalities.

6. Education of the pregnant mother and the family regarding pregnancy and childbirth. This should also focus on Common complaints of pregnancy, Nutritionand exercise, Emotional support, Adverse effects of alcohol and drugs, Benefits of family participation, breastfeeding, and Parenting

7. A system of regular antennal visits is to be informed, and the mother should be encouraged to adhere to it. Ancillary health support may be called upon, including family visits by the health visitor or assistant midwife. A monthly visit up to 28 weeks of gestation followed by a visit every 2-3 weeks up to 36 weeks and a weekly visit until delivery thereafter is desirable. Assessment of mother's health, including BP, weight, edema, gestational age, fetal growth, fetal heart tones, and fetal movements to be made. A more frequent visit may be indicated if complications develop or in case of high-risk pregnancies when the patient requires additional evaluation and management, including testing for Maternal serum al-fetoprotein, Herpes simplex virus culture, Hepatitis B screening (RIA), PPD, and if positive a chest x-ray is considered, HIV antibody if at risk, after consent

and counseling Ultrasound Scanning done when indicated. According to the society of Obstetrical and Gynecological Ultra sonographers, the indications for obstetrical ultrasound scanning include the evaluation of gestational age, fetal viability, placental location,growth retardation, multiple gestations, congenital abnormalities, breech presentation, post-term pregnancy, hydramnios, molar pregnancy or a pelvic mass.

Management during pregnancy includes, besides dealing with various complaintsand possible illnesses, The following:

A. Rh factor immunoprophylaxis Rh immune globulin is advocated to be given prophylactically during the antepartum period, after amniocentesis, after antepartum hemorrhage, and fetal death after postpartum and proabortion sterilization, transfusion of platelet concentrates and granulocytes and in a Rh-negative unimmunized woman after delivery of a Rh-positive or Du-positive infant.300 ug of Rh immune globulin is given at 28 weeks gestation in an unimmunized Rh-negative woman. Another 300ug is given after the delivery of a Rh-positive or Du-positive baby.
B. Dietary advice and nutritional support A weight gain of at least 11 kg during pregnancy is desirable for optimal fetal and maternal health. The weight gainshould be about 1-2 kg during the first trimester and then about 0.5 kg each week. Supplementary iron 30 mg

daily Folic acid 1 mg daily

C. Advice regarding lifestyles - exercise, bathing, sleep, and harmful effects of smoking, alcohol, and drugs are provided.

D. Emotional support and education about childbirth, analgesia, and breastfeeding are provided.

INTRA-PARTUM SERVICES FOR THE MOTHER

Cases of normal pregnancy and delivery can be easily managed at the secondary level of

health care or specialized clinics or hospitals, under-trained obstetricians withfacilities for investigations, and transport for referral centers if necessary.

The woman is encouraged to reach the hospital/clinic when labor starts but not to delay until there is a risk of delivery. In general, a primigravida is admitted when her regularcontractions are about 5 minutes apart. The multigravida should come into the hospital assoon as her contractions become regular. Rupture of membranes or significant vaginalbleeding requires immediate hospitalization.

The clinical examination includes the mother's vital signs and systemic examination, presentation of the fetus, the situation of the presenting part, cervical enforcement and dilatation, the presence of membranes, the pelvic architecture, and the distensibility of the passage. Necessary laboratory investigations are done,

Preparation of the patient, enema, voiding, and hydration are undertaken. Fetal heart rate isevaluated and monitored (monitored with electronic monitors, especially in high-risk cases). A pelvic examination is carried out at the appropriate time. Analgesia and Anesthesia aredone when indicated.

Delivery is carried out and completed under continuous monitoring in a standardprocedure. Psychological and social aspects are investigated.

The baby once stabilized after delivery following suction and clamping, and cutting of the cord, is given to parents for an introduction.

Complicated cases or labor < 34 weeks gestation are to be admitted to a tertiary level carefacility or referral hospital with intensive care arrangements and facilities for neonatal surgery if required.

The special services required at the specialized Centre are:

- A 15mt start-up time for the cesarean section
- 24 hours in-house anesthesia for obstetric care
- Shor term assisted ventilation for newborn
- 24 hours laboratory and radiology services
- 24 hours blood bank or its approachability
- Continuous fetal monitoring (with electronic monitors)
- Special care nursery

Regionalization of care of mothers, early recognition of high pregnancies and high-risk babies, along with the application of modern obstetric and pediatrics techniques, can go a longway to reduce maternal mortality and mobility and perinatal mortality.

POST PARTUM HEALTH SERVICES

Following immediate postpartum, including analgesia, perineal care, and psychosocial support themother is required to be given fluids and then a full diet. Early bonding and eye-to-eye contact with the newborn baby and breastfeeding of the baby are encouraged as soon as possible and then every three to four hours or ―on demand‖. The first few days are important for successful breastfeeding to be established. Care of the breast is essential. Caution is exercised in medications given to the mother nursing her baby. Rubella and Rh immunizations are ensured.

Early ambulation is beneficial in decreasing the incidence of bladder dysfunction andconstipation. Also, it reduces the chances of thrombosis and pulmonary embolism.

The patient, once stabilized, is discharged, usually 48-72 hours after normal delivery. Advice regarding diet, rest, activities, and baby care, as well as possible post-partum events, is provided, and follows up visits are arranged. Also, advice about maternal-infant bonding and family planning is provided.

Cases of a complicated pregnancy or delivery like cesarean section or breech presentation or ofany serious illnesses or complications during puerperium need to be managed till recovery in the hospital. Consultation with other specialists may be required. In normal cases, **4-6-week** postpartum visits are required to assess the return of the mother to a healthy non-pregnant state.

Clinic assessment should include breast, abdomen, and pelvic examination, BP, weight, Hb, and blood sugar. Thrombophlebitis, genital tract infections like endometritis or urinary tractinfections, or mastitis must be ruled out.

Baby is usually immunized against polio (1* dose) and Hep B. and advised to attend the neonatalclinic in a month's time

Checking regularly about the growth and development of the baby and giving immunizations on schedule is to be explained. Once a baby has been found to have no abnormalities at birth andat 1 month, there is little likelihood of developing treatable new diseases that a routine physical examination could reveal before the development of symptoms.

Mothers should be educated to overcome the anxiety and problems about feeding, sleep, and development. They should also be informed about possible infections and other benign illnesses and what to do about them, and when to consult the pediatrician or family physician.

ANSWERS TO QUESTION-4

REASONS FOR IMMUNIZATION OF CHILDREN

Several infectious diseases that result in considerable mortality, morbidity, or handicap among children can be and should be effectively prevented by immunization.

History is witness to millions of lives lost and innumerable persons in the capacitated year after year throughout the world due to many infectious diseases, notably smallpox, measles, diphtheria, tetanus, pertussis, poliomyelitis, yellow fever, cholera, tuberculosis, typhoid, and rabies. Some of them have been controlled or substantially reduced in incidence in many countries through immunization programs. Smallpox eradication (declared in 1979) was made possible through vaccination. WHO, through the Expanded Immunization program (EPI), is aiming the same for others, notably polio and measles.

However, some highly preventable diseases, namely tetanus, diphtheria, whooping cough, poliomyelitis, measles, and tuberculosis, still claim up to 5 million young lives every year, mostly in developing countries.

The resurgence of disease or occurrence of epidemics, even in developed countries where vaccinations were withdrawn or incomplete, such as pertussis in England and polio in Finlandare important warnings for keeping the vaccination status of the population high.

Certain diseases, like polio, rubella, hepatitis B, and mumps, even if not usually fatal, may result in serious complications and sequelae or congenital defects from intrauterine infections. All these result in considerable human suffering besides being a costly burdenon society.

Geographical variations exist in the occurrence of diseases either from environmental factorsor socio-economic conditions. International travel, however, can result in exposure and the occurrence of some of these preventable infections like yellow fever, typhoid, cholera, hepatitis A, and meningococcal meningitis.

Children, therefore, need to be protected from all those diseases through available immunizations, as required, not only to preserve lives and reduce human suffering butalso to save substantially in terms of the cost of medical care

Immunization can be active or passive. Active immunization is designed to use the specificmemory process of the immunological system of the body by antigen stimulation with a vaccine. The vaccine may be live, killed, toxoid, or genetically engineered. Now it is possible to modify the genome of a pathogen through site-directed mutagenesis to obtain safer and more immunogenic vaccines.

New vaccines are being developed for several diseases that are still at large and rampant or serious, like malaria, HIV, and Hepatitis C. Old vaccines are being improved for greaterefficacy or reducing adverse effects, such as pertussis and cholera vaccines.

For several serious diseases, short-term protection can also be provided through passive immunity. This is required along with active immunization or where it is not available or has not been or cannot be given for medical or social reasons. This is provided using specific immunoglobulins, normal human immunoglobulins, human convalescent sera, oreven antisera of equine origin. In certain situations, they are of immense importance to protect the child, either alone or in combination with a vaccine.

SCHEDULE OF IMMUNIZATION

AGE	VACCINATION
Birth to 1 Month	**1st HEP B** **1st OPV 1,2,3**
2 Months	**2nd Hep B** **2nd OPV** **1st DPT** **1st Hib**
4 Months	**3rd OPV** **2nd DPT** **2nd Hib**
6 Months	**4th OPV** **3rd Hib 3rd DPT** **3rd HEP B**
12 Months	**MMR**
18 Months	**Booster OPV** **Booster DPT** **Booster Hib**
2 Years	**Meningococcal meningitis**
2 ½ Years	**Booster OPV**
4-5 Years	**Booster OPV**
School Entry	**Booster MMR** **BCG**
10-12 Years	**DT** **Rubella for girls**
16-18 Years	**Td**

ADVERSE REACTION TO IMMUNIZATION

1. **NEUROLOGICAL**

- Convulsion occurs in about 1 in 1,000 cases. Prolonged convulsion occurs in 1in 100,000 injections in a normal infant after DPT and the measles vaccine.
- Encephalopathy - very rare – occurs in about 1-3 million. Most of them do notresult in permanent brain damage. They occur more commonly with pertussis than with other vaccinations. However, British National Childhood Encephalopathy Study could not say conclusively whether pertussis can cause permanent brain damage if such damage occurs at all.
- Paralytic Disease from OPV occasionally occurs, particularly inimmunodeficient persons.
- SSPE (Subacute Sclerosing Panencephalitis) rarely occurs a few years aftermeasles vaccination (1 in a million).

2. **LOCAL REACTION**

- Inflammation, induration, or a painless nodule is more common after the 1st injection at the site of injection.

3. **CONSTITUTIONAL UPSET**

- It is more common after DPT. Fever, screaming, or crying more than usual.

Persistent crying for more than 5 hours in the first 12 hours may occur after pertussis vaccinations and constitutes one of the contraindications for further vaccination with the pertussis vaccine.

4. RASH

- A maculopapular rash can occasionally occur after vaccination. It usuallyoccurs after 1 week of the measles vaccine.

ANSWERS TO QUESTION-5

NEED FOR VITAMINS

Vitamins are micronutrients in the diet which are essential to sustain life, promote growthand maintain normal physiology,

Vitamins act as cofactors in many enzyme systems and are therefore involved in different physiological processes, such as energy production and synthesis of amino acids, fats, nucleic acid, and nucleoproteins. They are classified into fat-soluble vitamins A, D, E, and K adwater-soluble vitamins C and are members of the B complex group. All the known vitamins have been synthesized. Availability of food depends upon the type of food, cooking absorption, and assimilation in the body. The deficiency of vitamins, which may be primary or secondary (to drugs or diseases), may cause serious consequences.

Fast Soluble Vitamins

Vitamin A (Retinol)

It is obtained from animal sources like milk, eggs, liver, and fish liver oil, and in the form of B-carotene (Protamine A) from green and yellow vegetables and yellow fruits. It is needed for the proper development of skin, bones, and eyes. It also acts as an antioxidant and is a factor in preventing the development of cancer. Vitamin A is necessary for the integrity of epithelial tissues and is involved in growth, fertility, and immune response. It is also required for the regeneration of rhodopsin or visual purple, a melanoprotein present in the retinal rods. Vitamin A thus influences dark adaptation.

Effects of Deficiency of Vitamin include Nyctalopia - defective dark adaptation Xerophthalmia dryness of the conjunctiva and keratomalacia boding to blindness Defective tooth enamel Keratinization of mucous membrane and skin Impaired resistance to infection Squamous metaplasia of respiratory mucosa Atrophy of germinal epithelium leading to decreased reproductive function.

Vitamin D3

It is obtained from Vitamin D fortified milk, margarine, and fish liver oil Cholecalciferol (Vitamin D3) is formed in the body on exposure of 7 dehydrocholesterol present under theskin to ultraviolet rays in the sunlight. Vitamin D regulates the absorption of calcium and phosphorus in the gut and their deposition in the bones.

Effects of deficiency of Vitamin D include:

1) Infantile tetany
2) Rickets in children
3) Osteocalcin in adults

On the other hand, excessive intake results in the calcification of various tissues, kidney stones,and the fragility of bones.

Vitamin E (Tocopherol)

It is obtained from germ oils of various seeds, green leafy vegetables, nuts, and legumes. Physiologically Vitamin E has an antioxidant property protecting membrane phospholipidsfrom damage by free radicals. It minimizes oxidation of carotene, vitamin A, and linoleic.

Deficiency of Vitamin E may be observed in premature low birth weight infants and is also associated with malabsorption.

Effects of deficiency of Vitamin E include:

1. He moly tie anemia in premature infants
2. Progressive Neuropathy
3. Posterior column degeneration- ataxia

Vitamin K

It is obtained from green leafy vegetables, liver, and meat. It is involved in the prothrombin infunction. Coagulation factors II, VII, IX, and X are vitamin K dependents.

Effects of deficiency of Vitamin K include_Hemorrhagic manifestation

Water Soluble Vitamins

Vitamin C (Ascorbic Acid)

It is obtained from citrus fruits, tomatoes, berries, and green vegetables but
cooking readily destroys it. It is essential for the formation of collagen, is involved in the integrity of intercellular material through the conversion of proline and hydroxyproline, andin the process like oxidation of tyrosine and phenylalanine, absorption, and transport of iron and its storage in bone marrow, liver, and spleen. It also enhances the conversion of folic acid tofolic acid. It is required for normal growth, tissue repair, and healing of wounds and bones. Itprotects many enzymes from oxidative damage by acting as an antioxidant.

Effects of deficiency of Vitamin C

Scurvy with tender bones and hemorrhages under the periosteum of long bones, gums, skin, and mucous membranes. Costochondral junctions become sharp and angular - Scorbuticrosary, swollen joints Wound healing is delayed Anemia from the inability to utilize iron or impaired folic acid metabolism Sicca Syndrome.

B Complex group of Vitamins

They are widely available from various food sources.

Thiamine (Vitamin B)

Thiamine pyrophosphate, carboxylase, as a coenzyme, is necessary for the carbohydrate metabasin. Thiamine is also required for the synthesis of acetylcholine. Thiamine is easily destroyed by heating and is extracted from foodstuff by cooking water. Polishing grains ofcereals removes most of the vitamins. Requirements increase in stress.

Effects of deficiency of Vitamin Thiamine

Accumulation of pyruvic acid and lactic acid in blood and tissues Impaired nerve conduction and emotional disturbances Clinically - it causes Beriberi - dry beriberi affectingmainly the nervous system, and wet beriberi affects the cardiovascular system mainly. In infantile beriberi, hoarse cry and aphonia develop.

Food Sources of Thiamine

Liver, meat, milk, eggs, whole grain wheat

germ, vegetables, nuts, legumes.

Riboflavin (Vitamin B2)

It is involved in oxidative reduction reactions in cellular respiration in coenzyme form. It has an important role in the mitochondrial electron transport chain and in amino acid, fatty acid, and carbohydrate metabolism.

Effects of deficiency of Vitamin Riboflavin

- Glossitis and cheilosis
- Seborrhea and dermatitis
- Circumcorneal vascularization with photophobia and blurring of visions.

Food Source of Riboflavin

Milk, cheese, meat liver, eggs, fish, green leafy vegetables, whole grains.

Niacin (Pellagra Preventing Factor)

It is essential in oxidation-reduction reactions and

mitochondrial electron transport.

Deficiency effects of Niacin

Deficiency is more prevalent in the maize-eating population. Classical deficiency disease ispellagra.

- Gastrointestinal disorder (diarrhea etc.)

- Neurological manifestations (dementia and muscle weakness)
- Dermatitis of exposed parts FoodSource_

Niacin

Poultry, meat, fish, liver, whole grain, green vegetables, and peanuts.

Pyridoxine (Vitamin B6)

As a coenzyme
pyridoxal phosphate,
Vitamin B6essential in
amino acid and fatty acid
metabolism

Effects of deficiency of pyridoxine

- Nausea and vomiting
- Hyperstability and convulsions in infancy
- Peripheral neutrois
- Hyperacusis

Food source of pyridoxine

Meat, liver, kidney,
poultry, whole grains,
fish,soybeans, nuts
vegetables.

Cyanocobalamin (Vitamin B12)

Deficiency causes impaired synthesis of DNA, defective myelin formation and arrest oferythropoiesis result in megaloblastic anemia.

Pernicious anemia (juvenile) results due to a defect of absorption or is secondary to gastric orileal disease. Food sources are meat, fish, eggs, milk, and cheese.

Folic Acid (Folate / Pteroyl glutamic acid)

Its derivation is concerned with the synthesis of purines, pyrimidines, nucleoproteins, and methyl groups. Deficiency results in impairedsynthesis of DNA in the bone marrow and intestine, causing megaloblastic anemia and diarrhea.
Food sources are liver, green leafy vegetables, nuts, cereals,cheese, fruits, beans, peas, and yeast.

Biotin

Coenzyme carboxylase, involved in the transfer of CO2, is synthesized in the intestine. Deficiencyresults in seborrheic dermatitis. Food sources are animal tissues, milk, and yeast.

The average daily requirement of Vitamins

Fat Soluble Vitamins	Children	Pregnant/Lactating
Vitamin A (ug. Retinol)	400-700	800-1200
Vitamin D (ug. cholecalciferol)	10	10
Vitamin E (ug. Tocopherol)	5-7	10-12
Water soluble Vitamins	Children	Pregnant / Lactating
Vitamin C (mg)	35-50	70-90
Thiamine (mg)	0.5-1	1.5
Riboflavin (mg)	1-1.5	1.5-2
Pyridoxine (mg)	1-2	2-2.2
Niacin (mg)	5-15	20
Folate (ug)	50-150	300-400
Vitamin B12 (ug)	0.5-1.5	2-2.5

MALNUTRITION

Malnutrition refers to conditions, diseases, or a state of deranged health resulting frominadequate or unbalanced nutrition, encompassing those due to excess food.

The Problem

Malnutrition is a major albeit indirect factor leading to the high infant mortality rates in developing countries. It also contributes to the high mortality of children in the 2nd year of lifein combination with diarrheal diseases and other diseases of infection. Malnutrition is the commonest cause of growth failure and pubertal delay. Chronic malnutrition during childhood results in stunting of growth.

Prevalence

According to a WHO estimate, about 1/3 of the population of children in Asia and Africaand about *1*/5 of that in Latin America have protein-energy malnutrition of various degrees, marasmus, and Kwashiorkor being the extremes.

While mild malnutrition is a very common problem in children in some developingcountries, for example, 70% in Nepal show stunting, the estimated prevalence of serve malnutrition in children under 5 years varies from 3% in Indonesia to 10% in Bangladesh.

Measure

However, real estimates of the problem are difficult to obtain given the fact that reliable anthropometric norms, commonly used to judge nutritional status, are hardly available in many countries. Malnutrition has been variously classified into 3 to 4 grades based on body weight as a percentage of expected weight for age (commonly by Harvard Standard) less than 60% being grade II by Gomez and Grade IV by Jellify

Etiology of malnutrition

Besides poverty, the main factor leading to malnutrition, various sociocultural and otherfactors involved include feeding habits and diseases like recurrent attacks of diarrhea, malaria, measles, tuberculosis, and other respiratory infections.

In general, nutritional deficiency diseases may be classified into primary or secondary. Primary deficiency is caused by inadequate intake of nutrients. High nutrient requirementsvisa-a-vis growth, early weaning, parental ignorance of post-weaning nutrition, and poor hygiene make the first years of life the most susceptible. Pregnant and Lactating mothers form another vulnerable group in the underdeveloped parts of the world.

Secondary deficiency results from factors or conditions impairing the absorption or utilizationof nutrients. Gastrointestinal diseases, impaired endocrine functions, severe infections, or inborn errors of metabolism may contribute to the production of malnutrition.

Diseases of malnutrition

Some of the specific deficiency diseases, besides general growth retardation and pubertaldelay, are:

- Kwashiorkor
- Marasmus
- Rickets
- Osteomalacia
- Scurvy

- Beriberi
- Pellagra
- Endemic goiter
- Pernicious anemia
- Iron deficiency anemia
- Xeropthalmia
- Dental caries

Diseases of malnutrition related to excess food or unbalanced nutrition, including obesity,diabetes mellitus, heart diseases, and hypertension though occurring worldwide, are more prevalent in the affluent societies of the industrialized world. They are polyfactorial in causation and are related to lifestyle. Specific diseases of generalized extreme malnutrition are marasmus and Kwashiorkor.

In marasmus, the child is markedly emaciated and irritable, and though the body weight is less than 60% of the expected weight for the age, he is alert and has a voracious appetite. Thefat in the adipose tissue is severely depleted, and there is muscle wasting,

Kwashiorkor

In Kwashiorkor, on the other hand, the child is lethargic and listless, and their appetite is impaired. There is marked growth retardation and edema of the dependent parts. The face is puffy, and the hair is dry, thin, brittle, and hypopigmented. They often suffer from diarrhea and are prone to recurrent infections

BERIBERI

Beriberi occurs because of a deficiency of thiamine (vitamin B1). Thiamine is necessary as acoenzyme co-carboxylase in the carbohydrate metabolism (Krebs cycle) for the conversion of pyruvic acid and alpha-ketoglutaric acid and is also involved in transketolase reaction in the hexose monophosphate shunt. It is also required in the synthesis of acetylcholine. Heating destroys, and cooking reduces, the Vitamin B content of the foodstuff. Polishing of rice removesthe covering of the cereal grain, which contains most of the vitamins. Gastrointestinal disease and liver disease decrease the absorption of thiamine. Requirements increase during fever and stress. Infants on breast milk of thiamine-deficient mothers develop infantile beriberi. It is seen in some southeast Asian countries where rice is the staple diet.

Pathology

Beriberi patients have lesions on the heart, peripheral nerves, subcutaneous tissues, and serouscavities. The heart is dilated with fatty degeneration. Generalized edema or edema of the legsand serous effusions occur. Venous engorgement may be seen, and the peripheral nerves develop myelin degeneration axon cylinders, beginning distally. The lesions in the brain consist of vascular dilatation with hemorrhages.

Clinical Manifestations

Early Beriberi patients have fatigue, irritability, apathy, depression, poor mental concentration, anorexia, indigestion, and constipation. Classically beriberi is of two types ofdry beriberi and wet beriberi.

DRY BERIBERI

It affects mainly the nervous system. The child is pale, flabby, listless, and dyspneic. Gradually peripheral neuritis develops with paresthesia, loss of vibration sense, ataxia,decreased tendon reflexes, and tenderness and cramps in calf muscles. Ptosis and opticalatrophy may develop. Muscle atrophy occurs. In severe cases, signs of increased intracranial pressure, meningism, and finally, coma develop

WET BERIBERI

It involves mainly the cardiovascular system. The child is undernourished, pale, and dyspneic. He has tachycardia, edema and liver enlargement, and loss of consciousness and convulsions may develop rapidly. ECG shows low voltage, QT prolongation, and inversionof T waves. Death due to cardiac failure may occur.

Infantile form of beriberi

It may manifest in one of three ways. The baby initially has vomiting, restlessness, anda puffy face:

- Cardiovascular type of a rapid course with dyspnea, cyanosis, and tachycardia.
- Neurologic type of manifesting as tremors and convulsions.
- Aphonic type with hoariness of cry followed by aphonia.

Diagnosis

Early diagnosis may be by finding:

- Low red blood cells transketolase.
- High blood or urinary glyoxylate.
- Clinical response to administration of thiamine.

Prevention

- A maternal diet containing enough thiamine, particularly in the rice-eating population, prevents infantile beriberi.
- Increased intake of thiamine for persons with a high carbohydrate diet.

Treatment

- Thiamine: daily dose of 50mg for adults and 10mg for children.
- IV thiamine for children with cardiac failure
- Other B Complex vitamins because the patients may have multiple B complex deficiencies simultaneously.

NUTRITIONAL EDEMA

Nutritional edema develops mainly because of hypoproteinemia with serum proteins below 2.5 mg/dl. It occurs from protein energy malnutrition (Kwashiorkor or marasmus kwashiorkor). This may be due to decreased intake or secondary to malabsorption or post-enteritis syndrome consequent upon recurrent or chronic diarrhea. There is intestinal mucosal damage due to sensitization to dietary antigens besides enteral pathogens. Milkprotein intolerance develops, and proteins are lost in stools. Hypoproteinemia due to proteinloss through the kidneys from various causes also results in similar effects. Infections like giardiasis, tuberculosis, hepatitis, helminthic infections, particularly hookworm infestation, etc., may also contribute to catabolism and anemia in the development of edema.

Edema signifies an increase in the volume of interstitial fluid in the tissues. Normally the dynamics of hydrostatic pressure and colloid osmotic pressure on either side of the capillary membrane are maintained in a way that there is a balance between the input and outputof fluid from the interstitial compartment.

Treatment

Treatment of nutritional edema involves:

- Protein intake is to be increased from the normal

requirement of 2-3 gm /kg

- Increasing calories intake through carbohydrates and fats. A protein-sparing effect isto be achieved
- Treating underlying infections enteric and other associated infections and infestations

- Treating anemia with iron

- Reducing salt intake may temporarily be needed

- In some cases, intravenous human albumin (salt-free) may be required to be given.

COMPLICATIONS OF UNDERNOURISHMENT

The nutritional deficit is a major albeit indirect factor leading to the high infant mortality rate in developing countries. It also contributes to high mortality in children in the 2nd year of life in combination with diarrheal diseases and other diseases of infection. On average, child mortality in the 1-3-year age group doubles with each 10% decline in weights below 80% of the weight standard. The prevalence of severe malnutrition varies from 3% in Indonesia to 10% in Bangladesh and Pakistan. In Nepal, 70% of children show stunting.The following are important complications of undernourishment.

1. Increased incidence of infections and their complications - particularly enteric infections measles, tuberculosis, staphylococcal pneumonia, Pneumocystis carinii pneumonia, and Gram-ve sepsis. Impairment of immunity occurs in several ways dueto malnutrition. The skin and mucosae do not offer effective physical barriers against infection.

2. Cellular immunity is grossly affected through:

- T-cell lymphopenia
- Reduced CD4 cell numbers
- Reduced CD4: CD8
- Reduce delayed hypersensitivity responses
- Decreased lymphokine production
- Reduced proliferative T-cell responses to mitogens and antigens
- Abnormality of the function of antigen-presenting cells. Impairedchemotaxis
- The defective bactericidal capacity of neutrophils
- Decreased T cell phagocytic functions.

3. Humoral Immunity

- Decreased complement activity, esp., C3
- Decreased IgA secretions
- Reduced antibody affinity

Anemia

Nutritional anemia is due to a deficiency mainly of iron but also of proteins, vitamin B12, andfolic acid.

Zinc Deficiency

- Decrease thymic functions
- Energy

Impaired cytotoxic functions<u>Iodine Deficiency</u>

- Goiter
- Impaired growth and mental development

Cretinism Vitamin A Deficiency

- Xerophthalmia Keratomalacia and Blindness
- Impaired resistance to infection
- Keratinization of mucous membranes and skin

Deficiency of Vitamin C

- Scorbutic changes manifest as bleeding from various sites - gums, subperiosteal,skin (ecchymoses)

Deficiency of Vitamin D

- Rickets in children -- showing retarded growth (height), rickety rosary, low legs, potbelly, etc.
- Osteomalacia in adults -- causing pains and tenderness of bones, malformation, and disproportion (cephalopelvic)

Deficiency of Vitamin E includes Progressive neuropathy and ataxia

Deficiency of Vitamins of B complex group

Thiamine Deficiency

1) Impaired carbohydrate metabolism
2) Impaired nerve conduction
3) Beriberi

Riboflavin Deficiency

1) Defective mitochondrial electron transport and various metabolic disturbances concerning fatty acid and carbohydrate metabolism
2) Glossitis, Cheilosis, Seborrhea, dermatitis.

Niacin Deficiency

1) Metabolism disturbances
2) Gastrointestinal disorders
3) Neurological disorders, mental impairment
4) Dermatitis

Pyridoxine Deficiency

1) Hyperacusis hyperirritability, convulsions in infancy, nausea, vomiting
2) Peripheral neuritis

Cyanocobalamin Deficiency

1) Impaired synthesis of DNA
2) Defective myelin formation
3) The arrest of erythropoiesis (megaloblastic anemia develops)

Folic Deficiency

1) Impaired synthesis of DNA
2) Megaloblastic anemia
3) Diarrhea

Biotin Deficiency

1) Seborrheic dermatitis

Specific diseases due to undernourishment of a generalized nature

Marasmus

Marasmus manifests as a markedly emaciated irritable but alert child with a body weightless than 60% of the expected weight for age. The fat in adipose tissue is markedly depleted when skin is dry. Muscles are hypotonic and wasted.

Kwashiorkor

Occurs due to protein-energy malnutrition, especially in a

weaning child who is listless and lethargic with severe growth retardation and edema of dependent parts of the body. The face is puffy, and the hair is hypopigmented, dry, and brittle. Flaky dermatitis and hyperkeratosis are often seen. Diarrhea and other infections are recurrent. The liver is enlarged with fatty infiltration. Marasmic Kwashiorkor is the term used to describe a child with a weight less than 60% of the expected and with edema.

Mental Handicap

Nutritional deprivation can lead to permanent impairment of brain development and mental handicap in the child, particularly if it occurs during the latter part of the intrauterine period and the first six months of life.

Nutritional dwarfing

If the undernutrition starts early in life and is prolonged, both the height and weight may be low, resulting in dwarfing.

ANSWERS TO QUESTION - 6

PROMOTION OF BREASTFEEDING

Both international and national organizations have endorsed breastfeeding as the optimal feeding for a healthy-term infant. In general, the percentage of mothers initially breastfeeding in developing countries is more than 80%. In the west, the practice declined in the present century as technical advances made formulated alternatives more attractive and acceptable. Currently, the practice of breastfeeding is enjoying a surge so that more than 50%of US infants are taking breast milk for at least some period. US Surgeon General has set goals of 75% of infants to be breastfed in the 1st week of life and 35% at 6 months. The trend shows that the first infant of an older mother with higher education is most likely to be breastfed. Given a healthy-term infant and healthy mother who wishes to breastfeed, there is little doubt that human milk is the best food. Its composition most closely approximates the need of the human infant. Human milk supplies not only the individual nutrients but also enzymesinvolved in metabolism, carriers to improve absorption, and hormones that may regulate metabolic rates.

Human milk also contains a wealth of components with immunologic properties that providespecific as well as non-specific defenses against infectious agents. These include:

- Cells like T and B lymphocytes, polymorphonuclear leucocytes, andmacrophages
- Immunoglobulins and other humoral factors, including secretory IgA, componentsof complements, and carrier proteins

- A specific antibody (especially IgA) and cellular immune reactivity against many respiratory and enteric bacterial and viral pathogens and ingested food proteins

Breastfeeding thus provides protection against gastroenteritis, respiratory infections, and allergic reactions. It is probable that altered microbial flora of the gut in breastfed infants iseven more important in protection than the antibody IgA.

In Japan, studies showed a fivefold decrease in the incidence of rotaviral gastroenteritis in breastfed infants. In other studies, though attack rates of rotavirus infection were similar in breastfed and bottle-fed infants, the frequency of clinical disease with diarrhea was significantly lower in the former. Similarly, it is found that cholera is rare in infancy, especially in breastfed infants. The precise role of antibody that blocks adherence of pathogens to the gut and the effects of other factors, such as lactoperoxidase, lactoferrin, and ant staph. Factor and lactobacillus bifid us and antiviral interferon are yet to be understood. It is possible that in the future, passively transferred protective components
in the human colostrum and milk can be targeted to enhance their effects through plannedmaternal immunization.

In addition, breastfeeding offers convenience: food stored at body temperature asepticallyand ready at a moment's notice in volumes determined by a feedback process, at least partially controlled by the infant. Furthermore, the act of breastfeeding offers a unique opportunity for maternal-infant bonding.

The maternal decision-making process is closely related to the social support and influencethat come from family members. The husband appears to be a strong positive influence. Prenatal as well as in-hospital breastfeeding advice and information are likely to be veryuseful.

LACTATION

Most women who wish to can successfully breastfeed. In most cases, failure to produce anadequate quantity of milk for the infant's needs results from failure to establish a suckling pattern that stimulates enough milk production. However, primary lactation failure also can occur due to insufficient glandular tissue, prolactin deficiency, or some other neurohormonal disruption. Surgical procedures sometimes disrupt ducts or nerve supply to thenipple, thus preventing successful breastfeeding.

Prolactin secretion by the anterior pituitary after parturition stimulates milk production by the alveolar breast cells. The increase in the volume of milk production occurs about 3 days after delivery. By this time, suckling, or if that is not possible, pumping, should be undertaken frequently, which stimulates prolactin production, consequently, milk secretion. Suckling also causes oxytocin release from the posterior pituitary, which acts on mammary myoepithelial cells resulting in milk release. If the breast is not emptied, maternal prolactin falls, and pressure atrophy of glandular tissue occurs, resulting in the involution of the mammary gland.

The quantity and quality of milk produced vary with time from delivery as well as from the beginning of a feeding to the end. Milk produced in the first five days (colostrum) is richer in protein and many minerals, as well as immunoglobulins but poor in carbohydrates and fat (energy content). By the third day, about 400 gm of colostrum are suckled in 24 hours, and then the milk production begins to increase dramatically. The infant receives a few calories in the first several days of life. In most cases, glycogen stores of the body allow a tolerance of this waiting time, and routine supplementation is to be strongly discouraged for its possible deleterious effect on the infant's suckling and consequent decrease in milk supply.

NUTRITION ADVICE TO PARENTS OF INFANTS AND CHILDREN DURING ILLNESS AND HOSPITALIZATION

The advice about nutrition to parents during illness and hospitalization of infants and children should address the following issues depending upon the age and condition ofthe child and the time available for details:

- The average nutrition requirements of normal infants and children foroptimal growth and development.
- The deviations from normal in relation to the morbid condition.
- Specific nutritional diseases or metabolic abnormalities need specialnutrition, like congenital lactase deficiency, glucose-galactose malabsorption, congenital chloride losing diarrhea, Hartnup's disease, Men key 's disease, and Bassen syndrome.

    - The information to be provided to the parents about the normal requirement of children should cover details according to the level of understanding and concern aswell as the seriousness of the illness and its nature. A broad overview of the need for different nutrients according to the age of the child in question in terms of caloric need and its different sources is useful. The benefits of breastfeeding shall be explained. It is essential to emphasize that besides varying grossly with age, sex, body size, and activity, the caloric need increases with abnormal losses of nutrients in stool or urine with fever, illness, and injury. Deficient intake is expressed in the individual child as inadequate growth, weight loss, or specific deficiency diseases or symptoms. Some examples, like night blindness from vitamin A deficiency, rickets from vitamin Ddeficiency, and anemia from iron deficiency, may be appropriate. Dehydration and nutritional deficiencies or malnutrition that may develop during gastrointestinal illnesses and the need for rehydration with ORS, as well as continued nutrition, are emphasized. Growth charts and their use may be illustrated to mothers for use at homeand to alert the physician if any deviation is noted.

Advice regarding nutrition during hospitalization

Life-threatening events.

Some cases of **life-threatening** events may be related to feeding, particularly in prematurelyborn infants. This may represent a maturational delay in the development of the suck-swallow mechanism. Usually, it improves with time unless significant brain injury is the basis. In older infants, such events are often associated with the transition from breast to bottle feeding.These can usually be treated by thickening the feeds. In more severe cases, avoidance of oralfeeding or administering nasogastric feeding may be necessary until maturation occurs. Occasionally **apnea** during feeding occurs because of marked gastroesophageal reflux.

Bronchopulmonary Dysplasia

They may require more calories for adequate growth than infants without respiratory disease. If oral feedings are not tolerated, peripheral parenteral nutrition, or more appropriately, central total parenteral nutrition (TPN), is required. Supplemented formulas can be used to increase caloric intake in infants who cannot tolerateincreased feeding volumes because of congestive heart failure or gastroesophageal reflux.

Necrotizing enterocolitis

Milk feedings, particularly hyperosmolar formulas, have been implicated in the pathogenesisof necrotizing enterocolitis in neonates. Also, neonates who were fed refrigerated, pasteurized, or frozen human milk exclusively developed necrotizing enterocolitis. Oral feedings should be withheld, and TPN provided. Advice is offered that in low-birth-weight infants 'oral feedings should be delayed by one week.

Failure to thrive

The goals of nutrition therapy are to establish metabolic homeostasis by correcting deficitsand replacing losses and providing enough energy and protein to promote growth. An infant who is below the third percentile in weight should be given a caloric intake higher thannormal to enable him to 'catch up in weight. The requirements in such cases may be 50% higher than normal or 150 Kcal/kg/day. Even a higher caloric intake may be needed when the infant's 'activity is considered during recovery. Evidence of significant weight gain shouldbe achieved in about two weeks 'time.

Malnourished infants often have anorexia which should be taken into consideration in feeding and dietary constituents. Malabsorption and other complications of undernutrition(like renal tubular acidosis) may need dietary readjustments

Inflammatory bowel disease

The provision of adequate nutrients is essential to make up calorie and protein deficits as weight loss is common for optimal healing and for prevention of deterioration in the patient's condition. Reduced voluntary intake due to anorexia and altered taste must be considered. Insome cases, continuous nocturnal nasogastric infusions of enteral formula through a soft silastic catheter may be necessary.

An elemental formula may be required due to malabsorption. For severe disease, when bowel rest is desired, parenteral nutrition is required through a central venous catheter. Bone age and puberty may be delayed, and sexual maturation arrested due to disease. They usually respond to nutritional therapy and control of the disease. Deficiencies in individual nutrients like iron, zinc, folate, or vitamins should be corrected with supplements.

PROTEIN LOSING ENTEROPATHY

Several disorders may result in excessive protein loss from the gastrointestinal tract. Some ofthe common conditions are celiac disease, gastrointestinal allergy, parasitized infestations, inflammatory bowel disease, enterocolitis due to various infectious causes, lymphangiectasia(impaired lymphatic flow)

Hypoproteinemia and edema are common associated findings along with other clinical signs of the disease. Anemia and lymphocytopenia may also occur. Diagnosis is usually by findingexcessive a-I-antitrypsin in the stool. Successful treatment consists of correction of the underlying condition along with good nutritional support in the enteral or parenteral form to provide increased amounts of protein plus supplements of various nutrients. Avoiding gluten in thediet (oat, maize, etc.) in celiac disease and allergenic food in case of allergy is to be understood.

Protein Intolerance

Protein intolerance comprising reproducible adverse reactions to a specific dietary proteincomponent is also called allergy, atopy, or hypersensitivity. It may present as a gastrointestinal disorder like milk-induced colitis, malabsorption syndrome allergic gastroenteritis. In others, it may result in urticaria and angioedema, respiratory symptoms, eczema It may be caused by cow's milk, gluten, or other foods.

Newborn infants absorb greater quantities of ingested food antigens than older infants or adults. Cow's milk protein intolerance occurs in about 5% of infant 's majority of whom show symptoms within the first 2 months of life, and this may continue beyond one year of age. Up to 60% of affected children may have a family history of milk intolerance.

Treatment consists of the elimination of the inciting protein, for at least six months, like cow'smilk protein or gluten in the diet. Soy formula or casein hydrolysate formula will be required.

COMMUNITY EDUCATION OF MOTHERS FOR RESPONSIBILITY FOR SCHOOL HEALTH PROGRAM

Mothers of school children have a pivotal role in the family's support for the education and health oftheir children and should be helped and guided to:

1. Know the various concepts and contents of health programs in school

2. Encourage and support the children in screening and assimilating the intended

knowledge and services

3. Cooperate with the school administration and the medical team in their efforts toachieve the objectives of the school health program.

A comprehensive school health program would comprise of:

1. Health services for prevention of morbidity and mortality from diseases anddefects through

2. Periodic health checkups and screening for early detection of any abnormality of physical, mental, or social health. Checking for vision, hearing, speech, locomotor, system, dental and mental health is a routine

3. Immunization programs

4. First aid and emergency medical care

5. Prompt referral for treatment of serious illness if any

6. Health education through the curriculum for imparting knowledge, motivation, andskills toward changing attitudes and behavior for health promotion.

7. Ensuring a healthful environment for health protection.

The ultimate objective is to increase performance and productivity and help attain a "stateof complete physical, mental and social wellbeing." The school health services, besides carrying out preventive and protective programs, aim at optimal childhood growth and development, also nutrition, learning disorders/mental retardation, child neglect, and abuse. It also participated in efforts to reduce childhood accidents and injuries and to control behavioral risks like cigarette smoking, alcohol and substance abuse, teenage pregnancy, and sexually transmitted diseases in adolescents.

Mother's responsibility is both supportive and persuasive. They can be of much help in informing the school health organization of any subtle changes in the health behavior of the child concerning, for example, vision, speech, sleep pattern, clumsiness, handling of objects, and in recreation, attention, or concentration.

On the other hand, mothers should keep track of the need for vaccinations as advised by thehealth organization. Also, they should inform the school about any contact with possiblecommunicable disease cases or visit areas of high endemicity of a disease.

Mothers should be educated to anticipate and cope with the changing physical, psychological and social needs and concerns of the children that occur with age. They can then provide a supportive, reassuring, and counseling role along with the school health team indealing with the problems, whether it be a physical defect, psychological stress, conflict, or social maladjustment. Mothers can also contribute positively to the success of the school health by attending the scheduled meetings with the teachers and school health staff.

PLANNING AND SCHOOL HEALTH OF HANDICAPPED CHILDREN

Planning requires an estimate of the magnitude of the problem. Handicap, according to WHO, is the social consequence of an impairment or disability. Broadly speaking, children who cannotachieve their full potential for physical growth and intellectual, behavioral, and social development because of -pathological limitations are

considered handicapped children.
The causes of childhood handicapping conditions are many. Many authorities attribute theseto perinatal complications. However, in some cases, perinatal complications and subsequent handicapping conditions may both be consequences of antecedent biological abnormalities early in pregnancy.

The handicap cannot be precisely quantitated because it depends on social attitudes and individual responses. However, disability and impairment can be estimated. The disability may be categorized as physical, intellectual, or emotional. Many cases have multiple disabilities. Thus, a child with cerebral palsy may have auditory, intellectual, and emotional disabilities inaddition to motor impairment.

Types of Handicaps

Neurological

1. Intellectual handicap (Mental Retardation)
2. Learning disabilities
3. Motor disabilities (Cerebral palsy, spinal bifida, brain injuries, residual paralysis afterpoliomyelitis, Hemiplegia, paraplegia)
4. Sensory defects (Deafness and deaf-mutism blindness, partial or complete include,including progressive myopia)
5. Orthopedic handicaps (sequelae of fracture, bone and joint infections, and otherdiseases like juvenile chronic arthritis)
6. Chronic visceral or systemic disease
    - Congenital Heart disease
    - Diabetes mellitus
    - Cystic fibrosis
    - Severe asthma

- Chronic renal failure

Planning of School Services

The planning is based on data about the number of different disabilities in the region and their severity, their effect on school performance, and any psychosocial adjustment. It alsoconsiders the vulnerability of the defect to therapeutic approaches, the possibility of progression, and the technical and financial resources available. With advances in technology and care, particularly for low-birth-weight babies as well as those with various congenital defects, there is an increased survival rate, consequently, an increase in thetotal number of handicapped children in the population. Although the trend is to integrate these children with minor defects into normal schools,with added assistance in some cases, many states have special health services for handicapped children. These programs have promoted the concept of team care, demanding that social work, nursing, and physiotherapy be included in the medical setup.

Contents of School Health Program for the Handicapped Children

1. Regular physical examination This should focus on the growth and development of thechild in relation to his handicap. Every effort should be made to enable the child toattain his full potential of growth and to acquire skills of a motor and sensory nature.
2. The diet and Nutrition of the child should be taken care of in the school by supplementary feedings, particularly in those unable to feed themselves.
3. Immunizations

4. Problems of adjustment at school should be taken care of in collaboration with the school administration. The child should feel fully accepted and integrated with the school environment, among the teachers and other staff, as well as among the peers. He should not be humiliated or given to feel inferior or neglected because of his handicap. Every child has the right to affection, love, and understanding. He should be ensured a sense of belonging and security. He should be given increasing independence within the limitations imposed by his handicap. The milieu of the child should promote confidence and self-respect. He should be provided with adequate opportunities for play, activity, and recreation and should take pride in his achievements. Appreciation and recognition of the achievement, however small, are necessary for the development of his self-esteem and the blooming of his potential.

5. Prevention and management of juvenile delinquency Handicapped children, particularly those with mild mental retardation and those with social handicaps, are prone to develop delinquent behavior. They may be exposed to an unsympathetic, insecure, and uncongenial atmosphere at home or school, and sometimes, having inadequate control over their impulse develops ungovernable, mischievous behavior and sex offenses. The school health team consisting of a pediatrician, Nurse psychiatrists, and social workers, along with teachers and parents, have a responsibility to help in the reform process. Special legal systems like juvenile courts are in vogue in various countries to deal with the problem.

6. Care of specific problems The school health teams, along with specialists in various fields, who can be consulted fromtime to time, will do all that is possible and practicable to ameliorate the specific defects and to diminish their impact on the total development of the

child. Many children have multiple handicaps. They need multi-disciplinary care.

7. Learning Disabilities may be secondary to mental retardation. Attention deficit disorder dyslexia, mild deafness, stuttering, and social moil adjustmentmay all contribute to it.
    a. Management options include psychotherapy, reassurance, and ongoing support, as well as regular speech therapy where indicated. Drug treatment to beused judiciously includes the use of dextroamphetamine, Methylphenidate (Ritalin), and Thioridazine

    b. Cerebral palsy Management is directed to the type and severity of the neuroglial deficit and associated problems, Prevention of convulsions (use of anticonvulsants). Physiotherapy is the mainstay of thecare plan Nutrition therapy, Occupational therapy, Special educational therapy, Orthopedic support, and vocational guidance.

    c. Blindness Braille the teaching. Other educational tools, Prevention of accidents, occupational therapy, and vocational guidance

ANSWERS TO QUESTION-7

DIAGNOSIS AND TREATMENT OF DIARRHEA

Diarrhea is one of the most common causes of morbidity and mort ability in young children,more significantly in developing countries. About 5 million children under 5 die each year in Africa, Asia, and Latin America, and about 10,000 in the USA from diarrhea. Each child suffers, on average, 10-15 episodes of diarrhea in the first five years of life.

ETIOLOGY

Diarrhea may be acute, persistent, or chronic. Acute diarrhea is usually due to an infection. The exact incidence of the causative microbes may vary from place to place and at different periods of the year. Nearly one-third of episodes of diarrhea are caused by viruses, rotavirus being the most common culprit, and about 50% are due to bacterial infections of the gut in developing countries, the rest being due to parasitic causes or non-infective causes, including lactose intolerance. Diarrhea may be a manifestation of infection outside the gastrointestinal tract in youngchildren or a symptom of another systemic disease or even stress.

Associated malnutrition and malabsorption, and any other factor reducing immunity, whethernatural or acquired, increase the problem manifold. A vicious cycle of diarrhea-malnutritionsets in because one contributing to the other, thus causing the heavy morbidity and mortality seen in such situations. Breastfed infants have, in general, a lower risk of infective diarrhea due to a wide variety ofimmunological protective mechanisms.

Bloody Diarrhea, compared with watery diarrhea, generally

indicates invasive enteric infection, lasts long, and is associated with more complications, and has a higher case fatalityrate.

Viral diarrhea

The most common agent responsible for acute infantile gastroenteritis in the world is rotavirus. A milder illness that affects old children and adults is caused by a parvovirus-likepathogen (Norwalk agent). Other viruses involved include Adenovirus, Coronavirus, Calicivirus, and Astrovirus.

Bacterial diarrhea

These pathogens usually produce toxins after adhering to the intestinal mucosa resulting in diarrhea

Mechanism	Non-inflammatory (enterotoxin)	Inflammatory (invasion)	Penetrating (invasion of mesenteric nodes)
Illness	Watery diarrhea Traveler's diarrhea	Dysentery	Enteric fever
Stool exam leucocytes	No	Polymorphs	Mononuclear

Examples	E. coli (ETEC, EAEC) E. coli (EIEC) Salmonella spp. Cholerae B Cereus Salmonella Spp. S. aureus Rotavirus Norwalk agent Giardia lamblia Cryptosporidium	E coli (EIEC) Shigella Vibrio parahaemolyticus Campylobacter jejuni Entamoeba histolytic	Salmonella spp, Yersinia entero-colitis Campylobacter fetus

Secretory enterotoxins e.g.by Escherichia coli (LT-labile toxin, ST-stable toxin - a, b) Vibrio cholera, Salmonella spp, Klebsiella, Shigella dysenteric, Clostridium perfringensNeurotoxin e.g.by Staphylococcus aureus (enterotoxin) Clostridium botulinum Bacilluscereus (emetic toxin) Cytotoxin, e.g., by Shigella spp C. perfringens Parahaemolyticus C. difficile A, B Enterohaemorrhagic E. coli S. aureus

Mechanisms and Examples of Enteric Infection

DIAGNOSIS OF DIARRHEA

Following a complete history taking, including that of travel, contacts, breastfeeding, and treatment were taken and a proper physical examination, particularly for hydration status, fever, signs of toxicity, and any systemic illness, an examination of a fresh stool specimen for fecal leucocytes and blood may be most rewarding for diagnosis.

This should be followed by stool culture and serological

and other studies were indicatedand possible.
Stool Examination

- Leucocytes — fecal lactoferrin test, microscopy
- RBCs orotidine / guaiac test
- Fat or meat fibers — Sudan stain, eosin stain
- pH testing — litmus paper or pH indicator paper
- Reducing substances — clinitest
- Parasites — Microscopy
- Culture — including on selective media for bacteria (Including sorbitol negative E. coli, and on Mac Conkey's agar for E. coli 0157:H7)
- Darkfield or phase contrast microscopy for V. Cholera
- Tests for the presence of toxins in the organisms cultured fromstools, GM, ELISA, etc.
- Electron microscopy for Rotavirus, Microsporidium
- Serology on stool or blood
- Sugar floatation or modified Kinyoun stain for cryptosporidium (in immunocompromised)

Other detailed investigations (were indicated for maternal diarrhea)

- Exam by Proctoscopy — for inflammatory colitis
- Rectal mucosal biopsy — for E Histolytica, granulomata etc. •
- Small bowel biopsy for Chron's dis, Whipple dis, Giardiasis,Tropical sprue, Lymphoma, Eosinophilic gastroenteritis

- Radiological studies — for Inflammatory bowel disease, Toxicmegacolon, Giardiasis, Pancreatic calcifications
- Breath test (C14 CO2) — for bacterial overgrowth syndromes(to detect bacterial deconjugation of bile salts)

MANAGEMENT OF DIARRHEA

Diarrheal episodes result in the loss of variable amounts of water- and water-soluble nutritive substances such as electrolytes, metabolites, and vitamins. This causes shrinkage in the volume of the extracellular compartment (EFC). In most cases, sodium and chloride are actively secreted from the gut mucosa and are lost in stools in acute diarrhea. In about half of the cases, it results in hyponatremia. With a fall of ECF osmolality, water moves from the extracellular bothe intracellular compartment causing further shrinkage of the extracellular compartment Dehydration, either isonatremic or hyponatremic type, results in various clinical signs like thirst, loss of skin turgor (elasticity), sunken eyes, sunken fontanelle, oliguria or anuria and shock depending on the degree of dehydration

PRACTICAL DIAGNOSTIC APPROACH

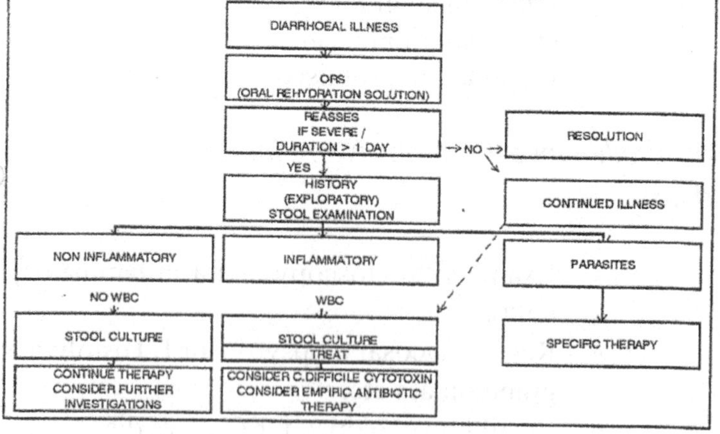

In about 5% of cases of diarrhea, especially if the child has

been given fluids with more salt, serum sodium level may be higher than 150 mEq/L, called hyponatremic dehydration with elevated ECF osmolality. Water, therefore, moves from the intracellular to the extracellular compartment. The classic signs of dehydration are less obvious. Irritability and lethargy occur early. The skin, in such cases, may appear leathery or doughy. Circulatory and renal impairment may result in all types of dehydration, causing thread pulse, fall in blood pressure, andoliguria.

Large amounts of potassium may be lost in the stool. Hypokalemia causes hypotonia of muscles and abdominal distension with ileus. ECG shows ST depression and flat T waves with U waves. There may be Hyper glycemia and hypocalcemia, particularly in hyponatremic dehydration_ Hypoglycemia may occur with prolonged diarrhea. With large amounts of bicarbonate lossin diarrheal stool, acidemia may result in deep and rapid "Kussmaul" breathing. Ketosis may occur with vomiting.

Management of Mild to Moderate Diarrhea

Fluid, electrolytes, and acid-base homeostasis should be preserved and maintained with Oral Rehydration Therapy (ORT). During diarrhea, while water and electrolytes are being lost, absorption of nutrients such as glucose, along with that sodium, as well as of amino acidsand dipeptides, is preserved in an enzyme-mediated active process across the cell membrane.

Plan A of WHO Recommended Schedule

Most of these cases can be managed on an outpatient basis or at home initially with any fluidavailable and preferably with oral rehydration solution (ORS).

Mother is advised to offer fluids that are easily available at home in as much quantity astolerated by the child. These can be in the form of Oral Rehydration Solution (ORS),

buttermilk, green coconut water, rice-based or other cereal-based fluids. Mothers should beeducated to watch for signs of dehydration and seek medical advice if no improvement occurs.

Constituents of ORS (WHO -UNICEF), in mmol/L - Sodium 90, Chloride 80, Potassium 20,Bicarbonate 30, Glucose 110. It can be prepared from NaCI 3.5 gm, KC1 1.5 gm, Sod- bicarbonate 2.5 gin (or trisodium citrate 2.9 gm), and Glucose 20 gm per liter of water.
Other standards or commercial ORS available have variable lower constituents which may besuitable for the maintenance of fluid and electrolyte balance and to prevent dehydration, particularly in situations where hyponatremia is more likely.

Oral Rehydration Therapy with Homemade solutions

Oral rehydration solution can be prepared at home using a mixture of 20 gins of glucose or 6-8 level teaspoonfuls of cane sugar (40 gins of sucrose), one level teaspoonful of common salt(5 gm of NaC1) with or without lemon squeezed in one liter of water (clean potable water).
Most soft drinks weakened fruit juices, or tea and coffee should be avoided. It may be possible to replace cane sugar with puffed rice powder or other cereals or cooked legumessuch as rice and lentil gruel or `Khichri' according to local availability and cultural preferences.

Plan B of WHO Recommended Schedule

Moderate dehydration or prolonged diarrhea may preferably be treated with a standard ORS (oral rehydration solution) and better in the hospital situation, under supervision. It should begiven freely till hydration is corrected.

Treatment of Severe Dehydration

The child is apathetic and moribund with parched lips, thy mucosa, absent tears, and markedlysunken fontanelle and eyeballs. Taken as a major pediatric emergency, severe dehydration must be treated vigorously to prevent complications and death from renal or circulatory failure or coma.

It is not necessary to give intravenous fluids in any but very severe cases of dehydration.Avoid overhydration and risk of infection through an IV drip. The volume required for rehydration = % dehydration / 100 x wt (kg) x 1000 ml.

Lactated Ringer's solution or glucose saline (0.45% NaCl/2.5%/glucose) may be started at a rate of 30 ml/kg body wt. in the 1st hour, followed by 20 ml/kg/hr. in the next 2 hours. Achild who starts passing urine in the next two hours should receive 20 ml/kg/ hr. of Ringer's lactate for the next 2 hours also. Also, ORS should be started concurrently.

However, if the child does not pass urine within 3 hours of starting the IV drip, provided he is fullyhydrated, acute renal failure should be suspected. In such a case, the fluid should not be pushed too fast, and specialists' opinions will be sought. Maintenance fluid is given as 0.18% NaC1 4% dextrose.

Potassium (3-10 mmol/kg 124 hours) is added only after the child has voided. As soon asthe child starts taking ORS and his condition improves IV drip may be removed and the replacement of continued losses done orally (ORS).
Hyponatremic dehydration cases should have rehydration continued over 72 hours to preventconvulsions by sudden fluid shifts.

Nutritional Management of Diarrhea Patient

Breastfeeding should be continued. Refeeding is to be

started early, and extra food (digestible) supplements are to be provided to prevent and correct malnutrition. Transient carbohydrate malabsorption may occur lasting for a few days, needing lactose-free formulas to be given orpartly diluted milk feeds in young infants only. Salted soups, bananas, etc., may also be suitable. In older children, iso-osmolar diets, like "khichri" milled cereals with small quantities of fats/oil, are provided in gradually increasing amounts at shorter intervals.

DRUG TREATMENT OF DIARRHEA

In the majority of cases of acute infective diarrhea in children, drug treatment has very little role to play. Antisecretory and Antimotility drugs such as loperamide may be of only limitedhelp and may, under certain circumstances, even be harmful.

Antibiotic treatment may be required for certain pathogenic infections. In general, antibiotics do not shorten the course of illness except in certain cases like cholera or shigellosis. They may be restricted to the following infection, used judiciously, based on culture and sensitivityreport.

Infective condition and Antibiotic

Shigella dysentery Cotrimoxazole 10 mg TMP plus 50 mg SMX / kg /D in 2 doses for 5 daysOr Ampicillin 100 mg/kg single dose or 50 mg /kg /D x 5 days
Enteropathogenic E. coli Gentamicin 5 mg/kg / d > Or Ampicillin Entroinvasive E. coli I OrCotrimoxazole
Vibrio Cholera Infection Tetracycline 25 mg/kg/d in div. doses x 7 days (in older than 8 years) Or Doxycycline 5 mg/kg / in a single dose Or Cotrimoxazole Or Erythromycin 25 mg
/ kg / d in 4 doses Campylobacter jejuni Erythromycin or Doxycycline Pseudomembranous Colitis due to C. difficile Vancomycin 20 mg/kg / d div. in 4 doses orally

Giardiasis Metronidazole 22 mg/kg / d div. in 3 doses x 5 days Amoebic dysenteryMetronidazole for 10 days

ADVERSE EFFECTS OF DEHYDRATION AND OVERHYDRATION AND THEIR TREATMENT

Dehydration means loss of water from the body, but it usually also implies loss or alterations of various ions. Most importantly, it results from gastrointestinal losses commonly in the formof vomiting and diarrhea but may also be caused by losses through skin, kidneys, and lungs or due to inadequate intake. Loss of intestinal secretions due to intestinal obstruction, fistulae,enterocolitis, or ileostomy are common causes.

Dehydration may be hypertonic when there is mainly water depletion, hypotonic when thereis mainly sodium depletion, or isotonic with mixed water and sodium depletion.

The osmolality of extracellular fluid (ECF) is affected by either intake or output of either water or sodium. Small alterations produce rapid physiological adjustments through the secretion of antidiuretic hormone, arginine vasopressin, by the posterior pituitary, Free water clearancefrom the kidneys is altered towards correction of osmolality. The volume of ECF is regulatedby the total amount of sodium present. A decrease in plasma volume causes an increase in thesecretion of aldosterone, which acts on the distal and collecting tubules of the kidney and enhances ionic reabsorption of sodium, thus increasing the volume of ECF.

Overhydration or water intoxication results when the excretion of water is unable to keep pace with the intake and production of water. It is found to occur in infants (due to adequate tubular function) following operations due to increased antidiuretic hormone (ADH) secretion, in adrenocortical insufficiency, or when parenteral hypotonic fluid is given in excess of requirements. The excess water is distributed between the ECF and ICF, causing a reduction in the concentration of plasma sodium and in plasma osmolality. Inappropriate secretion of ADH with the presence of reduced osmolality due to head injury or certain tumors may produce a similar clinical picture. Overhydration depending upon the degree and manifestations, is to bemanaged by a reduced fluid intake, particularly with restriction of water to about 2/3 of the requirements.

CLINICAL FEATURES OF DEHYDRATION

Degree of dehydration	Features
Mild (2-5% loss)	Thirst Irritability Dry mucosa
Moderate (5-10% loss)	Thirst Irritability Week thread pulse Loss ofskin turgor Dry lips and mucosa Depressed fontanelle Sunken eyeball Oliguria
Severe (> 10% loss)	Apathy/ lethargy, thirst, Peripheral circulatoryfailure (shock), Tachycardia, Loss of skin turgor, more marked parched lips, Dry Mucosa, Absent Tears, Markedly depressed fontanelle Marked Sunken eyeballs and pinched dry facies Anuria

In Hypermetric dehydration (Na+ > 150mEg/L), lethargy and irritability are particularlymarked and appear early due to shrinkage of the brain.

Associated hypokalemia, particularly in dehydration due to losses in gastrointestinal secretions, may result in hypotonia of muscles and distension with ileus. ECG will show STdepression, flat T waves, and prominent U waves.

Due to decreased renal perfusion from decreased plasma volume, acidosis and uremia may develop. This may be aggravated by lactic acidosis due to anaerobic metabolism at the tissuelevel and ketoacidosis from starvation. Kussmaul's breathing consequently results. Due to differences among compartments of body water as well as in total body water in children andadults, perfusion becomes compromised at a lower percentage in adults than in children.

Treatment of dehydration

Treatment varies with the degree and type of dehydration.

Mild to moderate isotonic or hypotonic dehydration can be managed with oral rehydration therapy. Oral half-strength physiological saline in liberal amounts may suffice in gastroenteritis. In general, fluids lower in sodium content are usually administered to infants.Isotonic saline is used in older children. Energy is provided as 5% dextrose.

WHO recommended ORS prepared from NaCI 3.5 gm, KC1 1.5, sodium bicarbonate 2.5 gm(or trisodium citrate 2.9 gin), and glucose 20 gm per liter of water provides sodium 90 mmol
/1, Chloride 80 mmol / L, potassium 20 mmol/L, Bicarbonate 30 mmol/L and glucose 110 mmol/L. It is suitable in most situations for the treatment of mild to moderate or even sometimessevere diarrhea.

Other standards or commercial ORS available have variable / lower constituents that may besuitable for situations where hyponatremia is more likely to occur and for maintenance of fluid and electrolyte balance. Homemade solutions (sodium sugar solution SSS) may be usedfor initial treatment at home prepared with 20 gm of glucose (or 40 gin sucrose) plus gm common salt (NaC1), preferably with a lemon squeezed, in one liter of clean potable water. Itmay be possible to replace cane sugar with puffed rice powder or other cereals, or cooked legumes, according to cultural preferences.

Treatment of severe dehydration

Severe dehydration must be treated vigorously to prevent complications and death fromcirculatory or renal failure.

Intravenous fluids may not be necessary except for very severe dehydration cases. The most suitable solution may be located in lactated Ringer's solution or glucose saline (0.45% NaC1 / 5
/ or 2.5% glucose). It should be given at a rate of 30 ml/kg body weight in the 15t hour, followed by 10 ml to 20 ml/kg/hour for the next 4 hours, provided the child starts voiding.Also, ORS should be started concurrently and given for maintenance. The volume of rehydration fluid required (over 24-36 hours) dehydration / 100 x wl (kg) x 1000 ml.
Maintenance is with 0.18% NaC15% dextrose (if required IV). However, if the child does notpass urine within about 3 hours of starting the IV drip provided, he is fully hydrated, and acute renal failure should be suspected. Fluids should not be pushed too fast in such cases. Specialists' opinions may be sought. Also, potassium 3 mmol/kg/24 hours is provided. It is added) only after thechild has voided. Close and continued monitoring is essential.

Hyponatremic dehydration cases are treated preferably with half or quarter-strength saline in 5% dextrose with a plan to rehydrate slowly (in 72 hours) to prevent the development of convulsions due to cerebral edema from sudden fluid shifts in the brain. The syndrome of hyperosmolality is usually associated with primary causes and uremia, shock, cyanosis, and feverand may love fatal. These infants are more likely to have been fed with fluids of higherconcentrations than those without hypernatremia. Elevation of chloride urea and potassium, along with hypocalcemia and hypo magnesia, is usually found. Renal venous thrombosis may develop Peritoneal dialysis may be required.

TREATMENT OF PERSISTENT VOMITING AND HEMATEMESIS

Treatment will depend upon the cause and severity of the condition of the patient. Many conditions of abnormal structure or function of the gastrointestinal tract may give rise to persistent vomiting with or without hematemesis in infants and children. Similarly, several extra gastrointestinal disorders can cause the same. Any persistent vomiting may secondarily cause hematemesis.

The following causes need to be considered according to the age of the patient:

- Esophageal disorders
    - Retroesophageal reflux/achalasia Peptic esophagitis Hiatal hernia Atresia of the esophagus Congenital vascular or mucosal rings, webs Stenosis Diverticulum and duplicationForeign body Maloney Weiss's syndrome.
- Stomach disorders
    - Hypertrophic pyloric stenosis Diaphragmatic hernia Gastritis Gastric volvulus
- Duodenal disorders
    - Atresia Duodenitis Malrotation Annular

      pancreas Superior mesenteric artery

      syndromeD. Intestinal disorders

- Atresia Meconium ileus Malrotation with volvulus Duplication Intussusception PolyposisCow's milk protein intolerance Gluten enteropathy Food allergy Hirschsprung's disease Appendicitis Strangulation of inguinal hernia Chron's disease Gastroenteritis Functional obstruction

- <u>Other abdominal causes:</u>

- Hepatitis Pancreatitis Gallstones Peritonitis
- Extra gastrointestinal disorders-
    - Cerebral anoxia Septicemia and other infections
    - Pneumonia,
    - Otitis media,
    - Urinary tract infection,
    - Meningitis,
    - Encephalitis Subdural hematoma Hydrocephalus Brain tumor hypoglycemia
    - Reyes syndrome,
    - Diabetic ketoacidosis,
    - Adrenal insufficiency
    - Renal tubular acidosis
    - Acute glomerulonephritis
- Inborn errors of metabolism Migraine Drugs —
- Aspirin Non- accidental poisoning Psychogenic vomiting Cyclical vomiting.
- Major causes of hematemesis include
    - Esophagitis,
    - Gastritis Ulcer disease,
    - Stress ulcer,
    - Bleeding diathesis,
    - Vascular malformation,
    - Duplication of Foreign body, including NG tube Maloney Weiss's syndrome,
    - Esophageal varices.

Treatment

Initial treatment consists of resuscitation of the patient and correction of electrolytes and fluid imbalance. Monitoring of vital signs and securing the airway is assured. Oral fluids will bestopped, and a nasogastric tube will be passed. Lavage and monitoring of hemorrhage are necessary. Whole blood and volume expanders may have to be administered. A CVP line may be necessary.

Specific treatment is planned and managed according to the cause of the problem, diagnosedby detailed history and thorough physical examination supported by relevant investigations. Hematemesis must be confirmed by ruling out the swallowing of blood. Any bleeding diathesis needs to be corrected urgently.

Investigations according to indications: Full blood count and platelets S. electrolytes and ureaXray Abdomen (plain) supine, erect Esophageal pH monitoring Barium studies Coagulation screen Infection Screen Liver function tests Metabolic screen Endoscopy C T scan head Rectal suction biopsy Toxicologic screen Arteriography Exploratory laparotomy.

Specific therapeutic approaches may include

For peptic disease

Therapeutic endoscopy, sclerotherapy, coagulation H2 blockers, Antacids Sucralfate bismuthVitamin K Surgery if needed.

For variceal bleeding / Extrahepatic portal hypertension

Therapeutic variceal sclerosis Vasopressin Seng took —Blackmore tube If no resolution —emergency portosystemic shunt

For vascular anomaly (superficial)

Endoscopic ablation

ABDOMINAL PAIN AND PROBLEM WITH WORMS

Abdominal pain in children is a common reason for consultation with a physician, but usually, tis a benign self-limiting episode. However, in some cases, it may be an initial manifestationof a serious underlying disease Causes needing urgent surgical treatment have to be differentiated from medical causes.

Abdominal pain in infancy

Abdominal pain in the infant is suspected if the child cries and screams persistently, is irritable and restless, draws thighs on the abdomen, and refuses to feed. Severe pain may present as asurgical emergency and be accompanied by vomiting, constipation, abdominal distension, or other physical signs.

Infantile colic

It usually occurs in infants below 3 months and presents as paroxysms of sudden crying followed by flushing of the face, drawing up of legs, and abdominal distension but without vomiting.The infant is thriving well. It may be related to feeding practices. Aerophagy, hunger, and immaturity of the central nervous system, manifesting as nonspecific irritability, may be the cause. Milk allergy is an unusual cause. Treatment is supportive until the colic almost disappears by the fourth month.

Causes of Acute abdominal pain

In most instances of abdominal pain, particularly in the older child, no specific cause is found. Itmay be dysfunctional abdominal pain, Constipation, and mesenteric adenitis are the most common medical causes needing symptomatic and supportive treatment. However, surgicalcauses, like intussusception and appendicitis particularly, must be excluded on an emergency basis.

Intussusception

It should be suspected in any infant aged between 3-18 months who suddenly developsscreening attacks of pain with vomiting. Acute onset of telecopying of the ileum into the adjoining distal segment results in intestinal obstruction.

The spasms tend to last 2-3 minutes and occur at intervals of 10-15 minutes. During each episode, the infant draws up the legs and appears pale and anxious. A-shaped sausage massmay be palpable, usually in the right upper quadrant. A few loose stools of small volume occur early. Later "red-currant jelly" stools may be passed. Rectal examination may show the tip of the intussusceptum. If not treated early, the infant may rapidly develop signs of septicemia and shock. Barium enema may show cupping. Plain erect x-ray film may show unusual bowel gas distribution and fluid levels. US Abd may help in the diagnosis.

Treatment of Intussusception

A gas enema reduction is the treatment of choice. Alternatively, a barium enema under fluoroscopic control may reduce the intussusception. Recurrence may require retreatment Peritonitis and septicemia are contraindications of attempted enema reductions, and surgeryis required. The patient is rehydrated, and shock if present, is treated as an emergency.

Appendicitis

The patient has a moderate fever, vomiting at onset, abdominal pain, distension tenderness overthe McBurney 's point in the right iliac fossa, and guarding in a typical case. Diarrhea and colicky pain in retrocecal appendicitis may be the only features.
Treatment is surgical and correction of fluid and electrolyte disturbances. Antibiotics may berequired.

Other Visceral causes of Abdominal Pain

- Choledochal cyst
- Intestinal Cholecystitis
- Intestinal Malrotation
- Meckel's diverticulum
- Volvulus
- Duplication of gut
- Strangulated hernia
- Torsion of testis

Medical Causes of Abdominal pain

Peptic ulcer

In infancy, gastric ulcer is more common, and hematemesis is the major presentation. In older children, duodenal ulcer is more common. Pain is periumbilical. Drugs like aspirin, steroids, NSAIDs, potassium chloride, toxins, stress (bums, intracranial lesions), sepsis, and shock maycause acute gastric ulceration.

Treatment

- Bland diet in the beginning
- Frequent small feeds
- Antacids
- H2 antagonists (ranitidine)
- Antibiotics for H Pylori, Ampicillin, or Amoxil and Metronidazole
- Bismuth preparations (Denel)

Gastrointestinal Allergy

- Allergy to various foods
- For cow's milk protein allergy, particularly in the first few months of life soy-based formula may be used.

Reflux esophagitis

Gastroesophageal reflux, common in infancy, may continue during later childhood, withintermittent symptoms of pain (substernal and epigastric), belching eructations, and vomiting.
Esophageal pH monitoring and endoscopy are required for diagnosis.
Treatment
112 reception antagonists Sucralfate

Fundoplication, in resistant cases

Treatment

- H2 reception antagonists
- Sucralfate
- Fundoplication, in resistant cases

Amoebic liver abscess and chronic dysentery

- Right upper quadrant abdominal pain
- The liver is enlarged and tender

Treatment

Metronidazole 20-30 mg/kg/day in divided doses for 7days.

Acute Hepatitis

(due to hepatitis A, B, C, D, E, F, G, or other viruses) Anorexia and abdominal pain, and jaundice are common Liver is enlarged and tender

Treatment

Hepatitis A is symptomatic, and Hepatitis B and C (chronic) may be treated with interferon.

Acute Pancreatitis

It is rare and may be secondary to liver disease or cholelithiasis or viral infection like mumps.

Treatment

Severe abdominal pain referred to the back, Vomiting, Epigastric tenderness with guarding, Correction of shock IV fluids, and Nasogastric suction Analgesics.

Passive Congestion of Liver

In congestive cardiac failure and constrictive pericarditis, pain, and tenderness in the right hypochondrium are salient features.

Henoch-Schoenlein purpura

- Abdominal pain is often severe and colicky and may be accompanied by vomiting
- Skin lesions over the

buttocks and legs (may be absent)

Treatment is symptomatic, often

with cortisone

Sickle cell anemia

Anemia with splenomegaly in the appropriate ethnic group suggests the diagnosis Treatment issymptomatic (hydration is important)

Chronic inflamma bowel disease

Pain may be intermittent with weight loss and fever, often without other signs.

Cystic Fibrosis

Abdominal pain from fecal impaction (meconium ileus equivalent) is episodic

- Bowel washout will resolve symptoms
- Dietary measures

Genitourinary causes Acute glomerulonephritis

- Pyelonephritis
- Acute cystourethirtis
- Acute salpingitis
- Torsion of ovaries

Other causes of abdominal pain

A few systemic diseases or those outside the abdomen may give rise to acute or chronicabdominal pain e.g.

- Right lower lobe pneumonia
- Diabetes mellitus with ketoacidosis
- Glandular fever
- Rheumatic fever and pericarditis, SABE
- Familial Mediterranean Fever
- Porphyria
- Abdominal epilepsy
- Abdominal migraine
- Drugs - NSAID and Aspirin • Iron

preparations • Erythromycin • Phenytoin • Sod.Valproate • Anti-cancer drugs

Recurrent Abdominal Pain

It is a common problem in older children and a cause of much anxiety for the parents andsocial handicaps for the child. Several organic conditions, as mentioned above, particularly chronic stool retention, gastritis or dyspepsia, food intolerance, irritable colon,inflammation, bowel disease, hepatobiliary disease, and Meckel's diverticulum, may cause recurrent pain in the abdomen. They need to be excluded by proper investigations.

However, most often, no organic cause is found, and psychological factors are involved in thepathogenesis. It is referred to as psychogenic or dysfunctional pain. Some of the backgroundand predisposing factors may be an overreaction to life events, family dysfunctions, disturbed parent-child relationship, too rigid discipline, over-protection, sibling rivalry, school phobia, and anxious and apprehensive or timid personality of the child who may show conversion reaction and complaint modeling. Management involves reassurance of the child and the parents, psychotherapy, and behavioral changes.

Problem of Worms

Worms or helminthic infestations are an important cause of abdominal pain. They are particularly common in moist geographical areas with low standards of hygiene. However, internationaltravel and contact with carriers can be responsible for cases anywhere.
The parasitic helminths may be classified as Nematodes (roundworms) and Platyhelminthes(flatworms) which comprise the Trematodes (flukes) and Cestodes (tapeworms). The common ones are discussed below.

NEMATODES

Ascaris lumbricoides (Roundworms)

Infection, which is acquired through ingestion of ova (in soil or food), may remain asymptomatic. Heavy infections can cause pain, weight loss, anorexia, diarrhea, or vomiting. Rarely the adult worms may cause surgical emergencies like perforation with peritonitis or obstruction of the small intestine biliary system, appendix, or Meckel 's diverticulum Volvulus orintussusception or pancreatitis may occur.

Larvae migrating through the lungs may cause acute transient eosinophilic pneumonia(Loffler's syndrome). Toxins from ascarids may cause chronic illness. Various allergic manifestations may result from roundworm sensitivity

Treatment

Any of the following anthelminthic may be used effectively:

- Piperazine -75 mg/kg body weight (followed by a laxative)
- Mebendazole - 100 mg twice daily for 3 days
- Pyrantel pamoate - 11 mg/kg single dose
- Albendazole - 400 mg (single dose or two doses therapy)
- Flubendazole – 200mg twice a day

Enterobius vermicularis (oxyuriasis)

Enterobius vermicularis (threadworms, pinworm) infection incidence is highest in school children. Prevalence is particularly high in populated areas in institutions such as mental hospitals. Threadworm infection is usually asymptomatic. The most common manifestation ispruritus of the perianal areas. Restless sleep, nightmares, bed wetting, and vulva! Irritation may result. Very heavy infections can result in gastrointestinal disturbances. Invasion of the bowel and appendiceal walls may occur. Mild salpingitis, cystitis, or urethritis may occur.

Treatment

- Mebendazole-single dose of 100 mg
- Pyrantel pamoate 10 mg/kg single dose
- Pyrvinium pamoate 5 mg/kg single dose

Treatment is usually unnecessary as reinfection is common. Otherwise, the whole family mustbe treated, and a second course is given after 2-3 weeks.

Toxocara canis and visceral larva migrans

Children ingest infective eggs passed by the infected dogs. The larvae get encysted in the liver,lungs, kidneys, heart muscle, brain, or eye, causing the intense local response.

The child shows varied symptoms with failure to thrive associated with pica, anemia, fever, cough, and hepatosplenomegaly. Brain involvement may cause convulsions or even hemiparesis. Intense eosinophilia is characteristic of Ocular toxocariasis and may present as granuloma or pseudotumor of the retina or retinal detachment Toxocara canis may also causevisceral larva migrans

Treatment

- Diethylcarbamazine 5-10 mg/kg for 7 days is effective, but several courses may be necessary.
- Thiabendazole 50 mg/kg for 3-5 days esp. for ocular cases
- Albendazole 50 mg / kg for 3 days

Ancylostomiasis (Hookworm infestation)

Ancylostomiases duodenal and Nectar Americans infections occur in most tropical and subtropical areas of the world with some geographical variations. With heavy infections, abdominal discomfort, especially after meals, and nausea and vomiting develop. Serve hookworm disease may results in profound iron deficiency anemia, hypoalbuminemia, edema, and cardiac failure. Development is retarded. Concomitant sickle cell anemia makes hookworm disease much more serious. Marked eosinophilia may be found after an early hookworm infection.

Treatment

Highly effective antihelminth are:

- Pyrantel pamoate 10 mg/kg single dose for A duodenal and multiple-dose treatments for N americanus
- Mebendazole 100 mg twice a day for 3 days
- Albendazole 400 mg single dose
- Flubendazole single dose
- Bephenium hydroxynaphthoate 2.5 gm— 5 gins
- Tetrachloroethylene (TEE) for N Americans 0.1 ml / kg

Trichuris trichiura (whipworm)

Heavy worm loads may cause abdominal pain and bloody diarrhea. Appendicitis may result.Marked anemia and weight loss may occur, resembling hookworm disease. Growth retardation is frequent.

Treatment Effective drugs are

- Mebendazole 100 mg twice a day for 3 days
- Difetarsone 1-2 gm daily for 10 days
- Albendazole 600 — 800 mg for 3 days.
- Oxantel pamoate 15 mg/kg

Strongyloids Stercoral

Heavy workload causes epigastric pain, bloody diarrhea, and iron deficiency anemia. Autoinfection is common and may be fatal in immunocompromised patients. Strongyloidshyper infection may be complicated by Gram-negative bacteremia.

Treatment

- Ivermectin
- Albendazole
- Thiabendazole 50 mg/kg two doses

Anisakiasis

Humans become infected when they eat under-cooked fish giving rise to intestinal disease with vomiting and epigastric pain with eosinophilia. Granulomata may occur. The most effectivetreatment is the removal of worms from the stomach by endoscopy

Trichinosis

A picture resembling food poisoning may develop during the early phase of infection. Later, encasement in muscle occurs. Eosinophilia is marked Patient may die of toxemia or myocarditis

Treatment

- Thiabendazole kills migrating larvae and early encysted larvae
- Mebendazole may be of value

Capillaria philippinensis and C hepatica

Abdominal pain with fever, eosinophilia, hepatomegaly, and epidemic diarrhea may occur

Treatment

- Thiabendazole

Tapeworms (Cestodes)

Important tapeworms causing human disease include

- Taenia saginata (Beef tapeworm)
- Taenia solium (Pork tapeworm)
- Hymenolopis nana (dwarf tapeworm)
- Hymenolopis diminuta (Rat tapeworm)

- Diphyllobotinium Latium (fish tapeworm)
- Echinococcus sp (hydatid disease)

Taenia saginata (Beef tapeworm)

In most cases, the infection is asymptomatic. In some abdominal pain with weight loss and eosinophilia, and allergy may occur rarely intestinal obstruction or appendicitis may result.

Treatment

- Praziquantel 5-10 mg/kg single dose
- Nicodamid (yomesan) 0.5 mg, repeat after 1 hour

Taenia solium (Pork tapeworm)

Most cases of taeniasis are asymptomatic. Diarrhea with eosinophilia may occur. Cysticercosis symptoms depend upon the site of the encystment muscle, skin, eye, heart, or brain.

Treatment

Praziquantel or Nicodamid are the drugs of choice as in T. sagniata

Cysticercosis — Praziquantel 50 mg/kg/day

In 3 divided doses for 14 days is effective

Hymenolepis nana and H. dimimuta

Heavy infections may cause

abdominal pain, diarrhea, and

osinophilia.

Diphyllobothrium latum (Fish tapeworm)

Heavy infection results in abdominal pain, diarrhea, generalized weakness, and megaloblasticanemia (in patients deficient in Vitamin B12 in the diet)

Treatment

- Praziquantel or Niclosamide
- Vitamin B12 has added if the patient is an anemia

Trematodes (Flukes)

Important flukes infecting men and causing abdominal pain are fasciola hepatica (liver fluke),Clonorchis Sinensis (liver fluke), and Schistosoma (japonica and mansoni spp) (blood flukes)

Schistosomiasis

- Treatment is with praziquantel (40 — 60 mg/kg)
- Oxamniquine is effective against S. mansoni (20 — 30 mg/kg)

Fasciolosis

- Treatment is with bithionol 50 mg/kg in divided doses on alternate days for 2 weeks
- Chloroquine is also used

Clonochiasis

- Treatment is with praziquantel 75 mg/kg for 2 days

ANSWERS TO QUESTION -8

TREATMENT OF CONVULSION IN INFANT

Convulsions occur more frequently in the newborn period than at other ages. In the preterm newborn electrical seizure activity occurs more frequently than clinically apparent fits. Theirduration is associated with poor outcomes, and they are poorly controlled in neonates by anticonvulsants. The incidence is estimated at 6/1000 deliveries in term babies and 20%
in babies < 2500 gins. The important causes are intrapartum asphyxia, intracranial hemorrhages, infection, and metabolic disturbances, including hypoglycemia, hypocalcemia, adhypomagnesemia. Uncommon causes include cerebral malformations, pyridoxine deficiency, and familial convulsions:

Investigations

Blood — Glucose, calcium, magnesium, sodium, and gasses. Culture Serology for congenitalinfections
CSF — Cytology, biochemistry, culture, virologic study US Head EEG Monitoring, if possible

Other special investigations, as indicated

- Urinary and blood amino acid estimation
- Organic acid Blood
- Ammonia
- Chromosomal analysis

Treatment

- Phenobarbitone - Loading dose 20 mg/kg followed 12 hours later by 6 mg/kg 24hours, given twice daily
- If seizures continue, an infusion of phenobarbitone is given at a dose of 5 —10 mg/kgover 15 minutes, repeated every 20 — 30 minutes until seizures stop

Clonazepam — is usually used as a second-line drug.

Loading dose 0.25 mg IV slowly than 0.05 mg/12 hours for the neonate. Continuous infusionmay be required with severe seizures.

Phenytoin (Epanutin)

Loading dose 10 mg/ kg IV slowly under ECG monitoring followed by 5-10 mg/kg/24hours in divided doses or as an infusion. Therapeutic level to be monitored.

Sodium Valproate (Depakene)

10 mg/kg may be increased gradually to 20 — 25 mg/kg per day.Useful as a maintenance treatment when phenytoin is not effective.

Lignocaine -

A useful third-line anticonvulsant in severe seizures resistant to treatment.Loading dose 2 mg/kg IV followed by 3-6 mg/kg/hour by continues infusion until seizures are controlled.

Paraldehyde

is given if seizures are intermittent. Rectal dose 0.1 ml/kg as a 10% enema in
N.S. or as a 50% enema in olive oil or Arachis oil. May be given MI (deep),

Diazepam (valium)

For immediate control of seizure. A dose of 0.2 — 0.4 mg/kg orally or as a rectal suppository. It may be repeated, if necessary, after 20 — 30 minutes. May be given IVunder close monitoring.

Other measures

02 administration if hypoxic. PCO2 maintained at 0.35 —

0.45 kpa Monitor blood pressure.Maintained a mean arterial blood pressure > 40 mnHg. For intracranial hypertension prevention and treatment, it is necessary to restrict fluid by about 20% less than the daily requirement. If full fontanelle, to give mannitol 20% 1 g/kg, if not oliguric

TREATMENT OF HIGH FEVER

Fever is the most obvious sign of the acute phase response to an invader. Active regulatory molecules, e.g., pyrogenic cytokines (11,1, LPN, and TNF), prostaglandins, and other substances (11-6, IL-11, etc.), are produced by phagocytes, lymphocytes, and endothelial cells.Fever results from prostaglandin synthesis in the thermoregulatory center in the anterior hypothalamus that controls the balance of heat production and loss. During infections also, exogenous pyrogens produced by microbes cause fever. The core temperature measured rectally or orally gives the true body temperature. Hyperpyrexia is the core temperature above 40 c.

The most common cause of high fever in childhood is an infection, particularly in patients under 6 years of age. It is usually viral, but many bacterial and parasite infections may also be the cause. Other causes include heat stroke, Kawasaki disease, collagen vascular disease, inflammatory bowel disease, diabetes insipidus, malignancy, epilepsy, and factitious fever (Munchausen by proxy). Hyperpyrexia is usually caused by exposure to extreme heat for several hours but mayoccasionally occur in infective illnesses, including malaria and pneumonia.

Treatment

Since hyperpyrexia can itself cause fits and irreversible harm to the child, rapid cooling is required to be done. The child should be bathed by cool water in a draught of cool air. The ice capis put. In less extreme cases, regular wet sponging or wrapping the child intermittently in a wet sheet followed by fanning is enough. Acetaminophen should be given 30 minutes prior tosponging.

Chlorpromazine 1 mg/kg may be given intramuscularly to reduce shivering and promote heatloss by vasodilation. This therapy is stopped when the core temperature has dropped to 39'c to avoid the development of hypothermia.

Acetaminophen (Paracetamol) oral/rectal 12 mg/kg or liquid brufen (oral) 5 mg/kg (max500 mg/day in children < 30 kg). It has a longer duration of action (6 -8 hours). Salicylates are avoided in children, except in Kawasaki disease or rheumatic fever, due totheir association with Reyes syndrome. Hydration with fluids should be encouraged as body fluids are lost during fever because ofsweating. Treatment of the cause, like antibiotics used judiciously.

TREATMENT OF MENINGITIS IN CHILDREN

Meningitis is commonest during infancy, particularly during the neonatal period. The incidence is 0.25 / 1000 in the normal weight newborns, while it is five-fold in those with < 2.5 kg birth weight. Meningitis may be acute or chronic and may be caused by infection (bacterial, viral, fungal, and parasitic), chemicals, or radiation. **Acute bacterial meningitis**may occur in the otherwise normal child or be associated with septicemia. It may result from the direct spread of infection from contiguous foci. Or compound fracture of the skull or infection of a ventriculi-peritoneal or ventricular-cardiac shunt. The single most importantvariable determining bacterial etiology is the patient's age. The most frequent organisms are encapsulated bacteria.

The commonest causative organisms during the neonatal period are E. coli., and group B streptococci, followed by

Streptococcus pneumonia, Staphylococcus, Neisseria meningitides,listeria monocytogenes, Hemophilus, influenza type B, Proteus, Klebsiella and other Gm-ve bacteria (which are more often implicated in neonatal meningitis than later in childhood). Multiple organisms may be involved in a single patient, especially in cases with a VP shunt.

During infancy, through 4 years, the common organisms involved are H. influenza type B (predominantly) followed by N. meningitidis (whose incidence increases with age), S. pneumoniae, Mycobacterium tuberculosis (more common in developing countries andimmunocompromised), Staphylococcus and Gm-ve bacteria. In older children, the main causes are S. pneumoniae and N. meningitidis, while less frequently, M. tuberculosis, H. influenzae type B, Streptococcus spp., Staphylococcus spp., and Gram-ve bacteria areimplicated. Rare causes include N Gonorrhea and Fusobacterium spp.

Clinical aspects of acute meningitidis

Most patients present with fever, irritability, and mental status changes, usually accompaniedby vomiting and headache, followed by the development of neck rigidity. Neonates and young infants may not show clear signs of meningism but generally present with nonspecific signsof systemic illness, which may include apnea and convulsions.

Though most patients are treated in the emergency departments, some will require intensivecare, especially comatose children and those with shock or fulminant meningitis or with abnormal neurological science or raised intracranial pressure. Similarly, those cases with a more serious illness like metabolic acidosis, hypoxemia hypercapnia, significant hyponatremia, and renal or liver dysfunction require close monitoring under intensive care.

Laboratory Diagnosis Lumbar puncture (if not

contraindicated, as in cases with raised ICP) CSF opening pressure, appearance, cell count, glucose, protein, chloride Gm stain Culture (bacterial viral, fungal, AFB) Rapid diagnostic tests Counter immunoelectrophoretic (CIE) Lactic acid (LA) Blood culture Blood/urine CIE/LA Tuberculin test, Xray chest CompleteBlood Count Coagulation profile Blood-glucose, urea, creatinine, electrolytes, bicarbonate

Specific Treatment of Meningitis

Specific treatment with antibiotics depends upon the causative organism isolated and the age ofthe patient. It is best delayed until the culture results confirm the cause. In the more serious patients and in many before the CSF culture and sensitivity are availableempiric therapy is instituted.

In the neonate, Ampicillin (150 — 200 mg/kg/day) is given along with an aminoglycoside (gentamicin 2 — 5 mg/kg/day or amikacin, 15 mg/kg/day) or chloramphenicol (50 mg/kg/day) _in divided doses. In the older child, a combination of Ampicillin (300 — 400 mg/kg/day) and chloramphenicol (75 — 100 mg/kg/day) or ceftriaxone (100 mg/kg/day) is given because in a significant proportion of cases influenza are resistant to ampicillin.

In those children with a petechial rash and when Gm-ve cocci are seen on microscopy, empiric therapy with penicillin 250,000 — 400,000 units/kg/day is started. Both meningococcal and pneumococcal strains are generally sensitive. Once the bacterial cause has been established, and sensitivity results are known, a single agent can be used if combination therapy is started. The course of treatment varies from 7 days for the meningococcaldisease to 14 days for S. pneumonia meningitis.
A short course of dexamethasone 0.15 mg/kg / 6 hourly early in the disease reduces the riskof hearing loss in H. influenzae diseases.

Treatment failure may be related to inappropriate antibiotics or complications like the subduralcollection of pus manifesting as the persistence of fever associated with a bulging fontanelle.

Nonspecific measures

- Fluid restriction to avoid SIADH in a well-hydrated child to 2/3 maintenance requirements with half normal saline and dextrose.
- Correction or prevention of hypoglycemia with dextrose.
- Supportive therapy- O2, Ventilation, ICP bolts, etc.
- Anticonvulsant therapy.
- Treatment of complications, if any.

TREATMENT OF NAIL PUNCTURE

A nail puncture wound in 7-year-old child should be managed from the point of view of pain,hematoma, and infection, including prophylaxis of tetanus.

The procedures involved are:

- Cleaning and washing thoroughly with antiseptics
- Pressure to stop bleeding
- Drainage of hematoma
- Antibiotic to cover possible infection with staphylococci, streptococci, clostridia, andother anaerobic organisms.
- Tetanus toxoid t ID according to the immunity status, repeated after 2 months if notalready given.

TREATMENT OF CHOLERA

Cholera is caused by vibrio cholera serotype 01 or V. cholera 0139 (Bengal). The V. cholerae 01, a Gram-ye motile rod, has two biotypes, classic and EL Tor. The V. cholerae 0139, isolated in 1992, is the new epidemic strain resembling El Tor, but it does not agglutinate with 01 antiserum, and its outbreaks tend to be characterized by the high frequency of secondary casesand a high attack rate in adults. Transmission of infection is through seafood (shrimps and oysters) other than through water.

Attack rates for cholera vary from 1-20 per 1000 population in different endemic areas. Since 1991 epidemic cholera appeared in the western hemisphere for the first time in this century, beginning in Peru. Case fatality rates in untreated patients may be up to 40% and lessthan 1% in the treated ones.

Following ingestion, the vibrio attaches to small bowel mucosa, multiply and produce severalenterotoxins, the most important of these being cholera toxin which activates adenylate cyclase through G protein, resulting in elevated cyclic adenosine monophosphate (cAMP) levels. This resulted in decreased absorption of sodium and chloride by vinous cells and increased chloride secretion by crypt cells.

Management

Rehydration of the patient, mainly through oral rehydration solution (ORS), is the mainstay oftreatment in most patients. Only less than 1% of patients required vigorous intravenous rehydration to prevent lethality. The following steps in management are to be adopted.

A. Step 1. Assess dehydration
B. Step 2. Rehydrate the patient through oral rehydration solutions except in case ofsevere dehydration and monitor frequently reassess hydration status.
C. Step 3. Maintain hydration replacing ongoing losses
D. Step 4. Antibiotic (oral) treatment of the patient with severe dehydration. This shortensthe illness

E. Step 5. Feed the patient.

Treatment of cases with severe dehydration

Patients with the following symptoms and signs have severe dehydration lethargy; unconscious or floppy with very sunken and dry eyes, very dry mouth and tongue, markedly diminished skin turgor, severe oliguria, or anuria, and (in older children) absent radial pulse and low bloodpressure.

These patients should be given IV fluid immediately using Ringer's lactate solution or normalsaline. While the IV drip is being set up, the patient should be given ORS orally or through a nasogastric tube, and this should be continued at 5 ml per kg/hour. Patients aged 1 year and older should be given 100 ml/kg IV in 3 hours, starting with 30 ml/kg within 1/2 hour, then 70 ml per kg in the next 2 $^{1/2}$ hours. Infants less than 1 year are to be given 100 ml/kg over 6 hours, starting with 20 - 30 ml/kg in the first half hour.

TREATMENT OF FOREIGN BODY IN THE NOSE

Foreign bodies in the nose commonly encountered in the emergency department among children may be animate like insects or inanimate objects like nuts, peas, beads, buttons, nails, etcThose of vegetable origin may cause a reaction with the nasal mucosa and may present with offensive nasal discharge, sometimes bloody. Irritation caused by pre-existing diseases of the nose, like vestibulitis, or the presence of thick sticky mucus in the vestibule of the nose may predispose to the introduction of foreign bodies by the kids.

Most of these can be removed by careful manipulation in the outpatient department. For others or impacted foreign bodies, a lateral x-ray of the nose and occipitomental view of the paranasal sinuses are essential in the management. Kilian 's nasal speculum may be used forgood viability.

A nasal pack with Vaseline gauze for a day is often required particularly if the mucous membrane has been scratched or bleeding has occurred. Antibiotics may be required if there is an injury of the mucous membrane or for a preexisting disease. Tetanus toxoid is to be givendepending upon the immunization status.

TREATMENT OF NOSEBLEED FOR THE MOTHER

Nosebleed (epistaxis) usually occurs secondary to mild trauma to the anterior portion of the nasal septum (vascular plexus in Kiesselbach's area) or on the turbinate (Rattle 's area), particularly if there is during of the nasal mucosa due to heat or fever. It may be recurrent insome cases and may cause anemia

Causes

The following local and systemic causes or contributing factors must be looked for andtreated accordingly after the initial treatment:

- Infections — Rhinitis, vestibulitis, sinusitis.
- Allergic Rhinitis.
- Bleeding disorder Von Willebrand's s disease, thrombocytopenia,Christmas disease, etc.
- Hypertension — Prolonged nosebleeds may occur.
- Vascular malformation — Telangiectasia, hemangioma, orvaricosities.
- Drugs – Aspirin interferes with platelet aggregation adhesivenessand may cause prolonged bleeding.
- Renal failure

Treatment

- Pinching the nose with pressure over the bleeding side for 10 minutes, in a sitting position, after cleaning any clots.

- If not effective, an Ice pack across the forehead may be applied, followed by insertion ofa pledged moistened with a decongestant nose drop, mesonephric 0.5 — 1% or 1% lidocaine with 1:1000 epinephrine or 1% cocaine, which is the most potent topical vasoconstrictor.
- Topical thrombin may be used, or a gelatin sponge may be put
- Cautery — electric or with silver nitrate or trichloroacetic acid.
- If crusting is present in the nasal vestibule, an antiseptic ointment (povidone-iodine) or an antibiotic ointment like neomycin may be applied.
- Combined anterior and posterior choanal packing may be required to be done by anENT surgeon.

ANSWERS TO QUESTION-9

INSTRUCTION TO PARENTS/COMMUNITY GROUPS TO AVOID DISEASETRANSMISSION

PERSONAL HYGIENE TO BE MAINTAINED

Maintaining personal hygiene and cleanliness is an essential first step in avoiding, catching, or transmitting a disease, particularly those which are transmitted through the oral-fecal route andthrough droplet infections. For example, many enteric infections responsible for diarrhea orgastroenteritis, helminthic infections, upper respiratory infections, skin infections, and infestations, as well as several urogenital infections, can be effectively prevented by observing regular proper personal hygiene.

Personal hygiene includes cleaning and care of skin, nails, mouths, and nose — hand washingbefore and after eating, toilets, nail cutting, and avoiding soiled or contaminated atmospheres or places.

FOOD HYGIENE

- Avoiding eating at unclean places — restaurants, and taking a cut or rotten fruit, etc.,from the market.
- Washing food items like vegetables and fruits before cooking or consuming
- Cooking food well before consuming, avoiding raw or uncooked meat, fish, or vegetables as they may contain germs or cysts of parasites
- Boiling milk or consuming only pasteurized milk
- Not leaving cooked food, especially meat, dairy products, or leftover food, unrefrigerated.

- Avoiding refrigerating thawed food items.

IMMUNIZATION

Keeping the immunity status optimal through immunizing the children and adults against diseases with vaccines at proper ages, as per the advised schedule, including boosters particularly for hepatitis B, diphtheria, pertussis, tetanus, poliomyelitis, Hemophilus influenza B, measles, mumps, German measles, tuberculosis (BCG), influenza, chickenpox, typhoid, yellow fever, meningococcal meningitis.

Travelers to endemic areas of various diseases should take vaccines according to thearea being visited. Pregnant women should take tetanus toxoid injections (as per advice).

AVOIDING CONTACT WITH OR ISOLATION OF CASES OF VARIOUS INFECTIOUSDISEASES

Period of communicability of various diseases to be taken into consideration. Avoiding sexual exposure and use of condoms to prevent transmission of infectionslike HIV, Hepatitis B or C, as well as other sexually transmitted diseases like gonorrhea and syphilis.

AVOID CONTACT WITH INFECTED ANIMALS OR THEIR PRODUCT OR VECTORS OFDISEASE TRANSMISSION

This is required to prevent transmission of diseases like rabies, toxoplasmosis, tularemia, leptospirosis, bovine tuberculosis, brucellosis, trichinosis, cysticercosis, echinococcosis, mad-cow disease (Creutzfeldt Jacob disease), etc.

Domestic pets like dogs should be regularly vaccinated against rabies. Vector transmissivediseases like malaria, leishmaniasis, typhus, yellow fever, viral encephalitis, plague, trypanosomiasis, Lyme disease, etc., should be prevented by appropriate measures.

INSTRUCTIONS REGARDING PURIFICATION OF WATER

- Storage in large reservoirs followed by chlorination by the addition of chlorine as I part per million of water. The amount must be adjusted to the water temperature and to theamount of organic matter present.
- Chemical pollutants, some of which may be carcinogenic, like benzene, carbon tetrachloride, and vinyl chloride, can be removed by chemical filters in the water systemusing activated charcoal.
- Boiling for 15 minutes disinfects water for safe home use.
- Small quantities of water may be purified by using chlorine, tablets, iodine tablets, tetraglycine hydroiodide (Globulin), or a tincture of iodine two drops/ quart of water, allowing contact for about half an hour.
- A portable filter may be used in homes or camps.

PREVENTION OF CYSTS IN FOOD

Several parasites undergo a life cycle with the formation of a cyst, which gets in the water or islodged in the food and can develop into mature larvae in the body.

Some examples are Entamoeba histolytic cysts in water, trichinella spiralis in meat,Clonorchis sinensis in the flesh of fish, cysticercosis bovis (Taenia saginata) in beef, and cysticercosis cellulose (Taenia solium in pork).

Prevention of cysts in food can be achieved as follows:

1. Purification of water
   - Sand filtration of water removes most of the cysts of E. histolytica.
   - Diatomaceous earth filters remove them completely. Chlorination of water in municipal water tanks - may not kill all cysts.
   - Treatment of small quantities of water with tetra glycine hydroperoxide (Globulin) tablet — one tablet per quart of water for about ½ hour contract or using liquid iodine,2% tincture iodine/ quart of water.

2. Proper personal hygiene and prevention of contamination of soil, water, and food withhuman and animal faces

3. Proper washing and cooking of fruits and vegetables, meat, and fish Cysts are killed above50'C by desiccation.

4. Keeping pork or beef at freezing temperatures below 5'C for 4 days kills the cyst cerci.

5. Control of imported meat and fish from endemic areas.

INSTRUCTIONS TO ORIENT SCHOOL CHILDREN TO PROPER HYGIENE

a. Cleanliness of the body is to be always maintained through daily bathing andbefore going into swimming pools, and after exercise and sports. Washing

b. hands at meals before and after eating to avoid infections to self and to others.

c. Brushing teeth several times a day, particularly after each meal andbefore going to bed — using fluorinated paste helps prevent dental canes. Avoid taking too many sweets and chocolates.

d. Avoiding exposure to harmful habits like smoking, drugs, and alcohol.

e. Avoid exposure to unsafe sex and learn to prevent getting infected with the Hman Immunodeficiency virus {HIV) causing AIDS.

f. Avoid visiting areas or camping at places, or being in contact withpets or persons likely to be infected with disease-carrying parasites likelice, ticks, flies, mosquitos, etc.

INSTRUCTION TO PARENTS / COMMUNITY GROUPS TO PREVENT WANT MORTALITY AND MOTHER MORBIDITY

1. Properly planned pregnancy and regular antenatal visits to prevent infections and other diseases and their complications. To ensure optimal intrauterine development ofthe fetus. Weight gain of 11 — 12 kg during pregnancy must be aimed. Prematurity and low birth weight of the infant must be prevented, and safe delivery ensured through organized prenatal care, which will also detect any genetic abnormalities.

2. Proper balanced nutrition of the mother during pregnancy and during nursing not onlyprovides adequate calories but also ensures the intake of optimal amounts of vitamins and minerals, which may have to be supplemented (like folic acid, zinc, iron, and calcium).

3. Breastfeeding of the infant at least for the first few months of life to provide him withthe required nutrition for optimal growth and development as well as to passively provide for adequate immunological defenses, both cellular and humoral. Supplementary feeding is to be given after the age of 3 — 4 months in addition to milk, and sometimes accessory minerals or vitamins are required. Gradually mixed diet in palatable form is provided.

4. Immunization of the infant as per schedule advocated by the health authorities toprevent diseases like hepatitis B, poliomyelitis, diphtheria, tetanus, and pertussis, and Hemophilus influenza B type infection. Also, vaccinations against measles, meningococcal meningitis, and tuberculosis in areas of high endemicity need to begiven during infancy.

5. Regular physical checkups of the infant to ensure optimal growth and development. Growth velocity is to be monitored. Any deviation from normal growth, feeding, sleeping, bowel habits, and acquisition of skills is to be corrected. Any diseases, whether congenital or acquired, need to be managed in time. Knowing some basic aspects of childcare at home by the mother or other care provider is to be encouraged to prevent illness and provide early treatment like the use of oral rehydration solution (ORS) in case of diarrhea.

ANSWERS TO QUESTION-10

INFORMATION TO TEACHERS FOR HEALTH PROTECTION AND PROMOTION OF THEIR PUPILS IN-PERIODIC PHYSICAL EXAMINATIONS AND SCREENING

Teachers have a very important role to play in the protection of the health of their pupils and imparting to them acquired knowledge and acquired skills for health promotion. The scope ofactivity for the protection of the health of school children encompasses,

1. Ensuring a safe and healthful environment:
    a. Cleanliness, including personal hygiene.
    b. Safe water supply and sanitary disposal of waste.
    c. Adequate lighting and ventilation in classrooms.

2. Give supplementary nutrition, especially to small kids, and prevent unsafe food consumption. Prevention of accidents and injuries:
    a. Removing hazardous objects, particularly in playgrounds and alleys
    b. Ensuring sound architectural designs and physical setup in schools, especially of the stairs and in laboratories.
3. Ensuring regular medical checkups and immunizations. Any child with acute illness shouldbe immediately referred for treatment.

4. Coordinating periodic meetings with parents and health staff (nurse/pediatrician), particularly in case of children with chronic or recurrent illness or any physical handicap likehearing or vision defect or any learning disability.

5. Encouraging healthful activities at school, including

first aid training, group discussions onmatters of health, physical education, etc.

Teachers have a central role and responsibility for the health promotion of children by educating the pupils about various aspects of a person 's health. This should form part of the curriculumat all levels to impart knowledge that will motivate changing attitudes andbehavior for health promotion. Armed with the required knowledge and skills, according to the age and intellectual capacity of the child, he will gradually adopt behaviors that will increase his health potential and capability to cope with challenges to health under adverse life circumstances.

Health promotion is any combination of health education and related organizational, economic, and environmental support for behavior conducive to health. Health education is the primary and dominant strategy in health promotion which is a broader enterprise creating asupportive environment for adopting a healthful behavior for self and society.

The objective of health promotion to be kept in mind is to ensure the child's optimal development as an emotionally and physically mature individual, with the ability to increase hisperformance and productivity for a meaningful and satisfying life in society.

Information to be given to teachers and community groups should consist of the following in simple terms and an illustrated fashion:

1. Basic human anatomy and physiology.
2. Heredity and environment, including diet, nutrition, and lifestyles.
3. Growth and development of children from infancy through adolescence, including thechanges at puberty.

4. Psychological and emotional needs for children at different ages, preschool, school, adadolescence.
5. Social adjustment problems in relation to teachers, peers, and parents of children, particularly in those from problem families or broken homes. Specific problems likeparent-child adjustment enuresis delinquency, Hyperactivity, Attention deficit disorder, etc., are to be discussed.
6. Special problems like sexual maturation and perversions, contraception, engaging in pregnancy, family life, and drug and alcohol abuse should be explained to teachers.
7. Organizations, services, support resources, and legislations existing or in vogue for health promotion activities and for dealing with specific problems should be broughtto their notice to take advantage of in making a child into a responsible, useful adult.

CONCLUSION

The above information is never a substitute for professional medical advice and treatment. Seek medical help immediately in case of an emergency.

References:

1. Billiamin A. Alli, (n.d.). National Center for Biotechnology Information. https://www.ncbi.nlm.nih.gov/pmc/articles/PMC2536916/pdf/jnma00009-0039.pdf
2. Billiamin A. Alli, (n.d.). National Center for Biotechnology Information. https://www.ncbi.nlm.nih.gov/pmc/articles/PMC2537146/pdf/jnma00017-0059.pdf

Made in the USA
Monee, IL
13 May 2025

17411784R00069